Advance Praise for Just Breathe

"Brilliantly told, compelling, heartfelt, and beautiful. Just Breathe *is a powerful read."*

—Robert J. Sawyer, Hugo Award-winning author of *Calculating God*

"This is a book written from the heart—a gallant heart full of courage, hope, and the love of life. It provides uncommon insight into what, unfortunately, is an all too common experience. Stephen King's account of his life as a cancer patient is, like the man himself, honest and compassionate."

—Suzanne North, author of *Bones To Pick*

"Stephen is a beautiful, open, and friendly man who walked up to me in a mall to ask when my next book would be published. As I've come to know him better, I've realised he has quite the story to tell himself. This is that story. And you can add courage and generosity to the list of attributes."

—Nalo Hopkinson, author of *The Salt Roads*

"Stephen Graham King writes in a way that transcends the traditional reader-writer relationship. You don't read this book so much as you stand beside the author, his arm around your shoulder, as he lets you in on the intimate thoughts, feelings, and emotions he experienced through his trials. His words are honest, touching, poignant, and heartfelt. They come alive like a dear friend sharing his story across a coffee shop table."

—Mark Leslie, author of *One Hand Screaming*

JUST BREATHE

JUST BREATHE

✦

My Journey Through Cancer and Back

Stephen Graham King

iUniverse, Inc.
New York Lincoln Shanghai

JUST BREATHE
My Journey Through Cancer and Back

iUniverse books may be ordered through booksellers or by contacting:

iUniverse
2021 Pine Lake Road, Suite 100
Lincoln, NE 68512
www.iuniverse.com
1-800-Authors (1-800-288-4677)

Cover photograph by Debra Marshall
Author Photo by David Findlay

ISBN-13: 978-0-595-37530-1 (pbk)
ISBN-13: 978-0-595-81923-2 (ebk)
ISBN-10: 0-595-37530-8 (pbk)
ISBN-10: 0-595-81923-0 (ebk)

Printed in the United States of America

This is for my parents, Ray and Eve, who not only gave me life, but also the spirit to live it and the will to fight for it.

Who would have thought when chance came calling
that this would be my defining story
and who could have guessed on my life's journey
I could find my way through this extraordinary day

"Extraordinary Day"
by Delta Goodrem

Contents

One
To Begin at the Beginning...?

All stories have a beginning, middle, and end. That's the common wisdom, right? As a writer, I agree. I create characters and take them from an initial event, guide them through a series of hoops, and see what they do. As I write them, I see how they react to the situations and how the situations change them. The scenario plays out and comes to its logical conclusion. The End...fade out...closing credits.

But that isn't life, is it?

Like points on a curve, life is far more slippery and impossible to pigeonhole. What is the initial event? Where does a circle begin? Like a homemade Moebius loop, take a strip of paper, twist it once, and glue the front of one end to the back of the other. Try finding the beginning then.

As a person who has lived through cancer, I have lost that sense of beginning, middle, and end. Does my war against cancer begin with the diagnosis? The disease had been in my body for a long time before that. Does it begin with the first injury to that knee so many years ago?

Any attempt to establish that initial point boggles the mind. If I could freeze time with some kind of magic lens, that is, focus on that nanosecond when the cells mutated and became malignant, maybe. But that mutation was caused by something else, an injury or some unknown environmental cause. The chain stretches into the past, each link connecting multiple events.

It's rare we recognize the moments that will change our lives in the instant they are occurring. So, to tell the story of my cancer, the disease that would so radically alter my body and my mind, my heart and my soul, I have no choice but to be arbitrary. I'm just picking a point and claiming it, planting my flag in the mountain. X marks the spot. You are here.

When the year 2000 arrived, I was on the verge of my thirty-seventh birthday. I remember pondering that particular birthday in high school. It seemed I would be irretrievably old when the turn of the century came. As it happened, I had been living in Toronto for two years; having moved there with the man I thought I would share my life with. I was working for Coles (the Book People), which was then owned by Chapters, but has since become part of Indigo. I had been lucky enough to be hired for a full-time position with the Eaton Centre store barely a month after arriving and was made assistant manager a year later. I spent my days surrounded by books and other book lovers. I had benefits and a good group of people to work with. But, as they must, things changed. Six months after arriving in Toronto, my partner and I were living apart. Six months after that, it was over.

To complicate things further, we had just signed the lease on a new apartment with a mutual friend. We were left struggling to build a friendship from the remains of our relationship in the same house. If a similar situation ever arises for you, don't do it. Regardless of the reasons, it's a bad idea. To be fair, I was glad of Kerry's presence many times. I had yet to find a social groove in Toronto. I knew few people, and I was close to fewer still. Coming from a city that was smaller and, in some ways, friendlier, where I had spent eighteen years building relationships, the unwanted solitude was hard.

I took solace in work, in my place as second-in-command of my store. Then, one day, I bumped my knee into a stack of books piled on a bargain book pyramid and nearly passed out from the pain.

I've had problems with my left knee for most of my adult life. We don't have good joints in my family to begin with, and an injury worsened mine at university. I was appearing in a play for my fourth-year acting class, *The Persecution and Assassination of Jean-Paul Marat as Performed by the Inmates at the Asylum at Charenton under the Direction of the Marquis de Sade*, mercifully shortened in conversation to the *Marat/Sade*. The play was extremely physical. My one main speech was about man being a mad animal. I spent most of my time crouched near the floor. Sometime during the rehearsals, my left knee popped out and back in. I only discovered this after my knee was sore for a week and I went to the Student Health Centre to have it checked. Being young and foolish, I didn't do the exercises the physiotherapist prescribed. Over time, the problem worsened until about seven years ago. A new round of physiotherapy and visits to my doctor led to an arthroscopy. With a tiny camera inserted in the joint, the orthopaedist found and removed osteophytes (small, lumpy bone growths) from the back of my kneecap. Once I healed from the procedure, I noticed a marked improvement, but, as before, the weakened joint was always a source of trouble. Whenever I slipped or stumbled (on ice or stairs), the stress always went onto this joint. A bad stumble in the winter of 1998–1999 started an entirely new cycle of pain and swelling. Gradually, the joint reweakened and needed constant wrapping. My ex had a doctor he really liked, Dr. Peter Satok, and he encouraged me to see him. I was due for a checkup, but, being me, I repeatedly put it off. A painful slip in the bathroom finally broke my stubbornness and hesitance, and I finally went to see him for the first time. That checkup started what I soon called my *Magical Medical Tour*. (Coming soon to a doctor's office near you!) It eventually changed everything.

For my sore knee was, in fact, the result of a synovial sarcoma, a rare soft tissue cancer that tends to strike young men who are either tall or long-boned. My chances of winning the lottery were better.

We all know about cancer. Every day, pink ribbons and yellow daffodils confront us. Ads for self-examination or encouraging us to give blood as well as stories of a new celebrity stricken with the disease fill our TV screens. It seems we all know someone or someone who knows someone who has been stricken with cancer and has either survived or died. We know basically what the disease is. Something, some combination of genetics and environment, causes a cell to mutate into a new, virulent form. This new cell grows, destroys the cells around it, and replaces them with copies of itself. Left unchecked, the disease eats away at breast, muscle, bone, or tissue. One of cancer's great mysteries is the way some rare cases just go away. However, in far too many cases, cancer kills, and we barely understand why.

Of course, there are treatments, mainstream and fringe. I don't pretend to know the success rate of fringe therapies. A well-meaning friend suggested some to me, but I like evidence, studies, and published results. Someone who said they knew someone who cured themselves with herbs wasn't enough for me to gamble my life. However, if you choose mainstream cancer therapies, as I did, you are consigned to a brutal path. Despite the diagnostic tools at our disposal, modern cancer treatment is barbaric, something akin to a medieval torture chamber.

There are three basic courses of action:

- Radiation: attack the tumour with a lesser version of the power that levelled Hiroshima and burned millions of lives to ash

- Chemotherapy: poison the tumour with drugs that kill the cancer and take hair follicles, mucous membranes, and white blood cells with it

- Surgery: cut away the diseased cells and a shell of healthy tissue around them

These are the options. The man who first spoke of cancer treatment to me in these brutal terms had lost his partner to a short, ugly battle with lymphoma and spoke the allusion with understandable bitterness in his voice. When I think of the harshness of the weapons used against my cancer, it doesn't speak to me of the medical community's inadequacies. It speaks to me of the devastating, ruthless power this disease holds over us. We are meeting the enemy with the only weapons we have that match it.

Through the course of my cancer, I experienced all three of these weapons arrayed against the rogue cells invading me. I lost my hair in addition to my ability to normally walk up a flight of stairs or dance. On some of the darkest days, I even lost my will to continue fighting. My hair came back, and my will to fight the disease returned. The dancing and the stairs are gone for good.

But like the yin and yang, if I had never become ill, there are people I would have never met. Some are health care professionals whose skills and compassion I will forever hold in awe. Some are just admirable people with kind hearts and loving souls who have crossed my path and shone light into the dark corners.

At one point, Peter told me this experience would be a magnifier. Peoples' strengths and weaknesses would stand out, shadowed in high-contrast black and white. At the time I thought he was only referencing others, but it would prove true of me as well. If it weren't for the disease, I might have never seen the depth of my own strength or appreciated the depth of my friends' love.

For most of my adult life, I have written—science fiction novels, journals, letters, and my Web site. My constant scribblings have helped me sift through the chaos in my head. This story has burned in me, sometimes a hole like the pinpoint of a laser and sometimes like slow, glowing embers. But I need to write it to understand, that is, to peel away the layers of the onion and see what—if anything—can be gleaned from this horror. We don't talk about disease in our culture. We turn it into maudlin movies of the week, but we don't talk about its effects or the toll it takes. People think they are intruding if they ask questions.

So many times, someone would ask if I minded talking about it. A part of me wanted to scream, "Of course I want to talk about it!" It was real. It happened.

We must talk about it in order to air the truths hidden from view and honour those that work to help people through it. To do these things, we, the people who have battled these illnesses, must tell our stories loudly and to all who will listen. I don't pretend to have the answers or know what you should do if confronted with something similar. This is just the story of how I travelled from there to here: my path and how I walked it.

But to start, we must pick a point on the curve and find a place to begin. We must open the curtain and join the scene of a life already in progress. This is where we plant the flag.

You are here.

Two
Me

To know the fight, one must first know the fighter.

I was born April 6, 1963, in the Providence Hospital in Moose Jaw, Saskatchewan. Years later, after fifteen years of friendship, I discovered my best friend, Gordon, was born there—six days after me.

If you have never visited the prairies, you must. People will tell you there is nothing of interest there; it's nothing but flat space. Look beyond the emptiness to see something else, something primal in a sky that spreads around you in all directions along with the amber gold of wheat fields that ripple when the wind comes up, like muscles under skin.

One time in Toronto, I was having a bad day. Feeling lost and alone in the city, I was uncertain of why I was here and why I didn't just pack up and go home. I left the house and began walking east along Queen Street, wandering until I hit the Beaches. On a whim, I walked down to the shore of Lake Ontario. As soon as I hit the boardwalk and saw that sky, without any CN Tower or skyscrapers or anything between it and me, all the sadness and homesickness flew out of me in one great gust of outgoing breath. That unhindered sky said, "It's okay. Let me have it. You don't need it anymore."

My parents, Raymond Leslie Norman and Dorothy Evelyn, emigrated from England with my oldest sister, Susan, in 1950 to the land of endless prairie skies. They followed my father's mother and sister, who had arrived two years earlier. I have always been tickled by the fact that they married when my mother was twenty-six and my father was nineteen. My paternal grandfather's death, their wedding, and granddad's funeral happened in the space of a week and on the heels of World War II in England. I guess marching to the beat of your own drummer runs in the genes.

Hardship was no stranger to them in England or Canada. During the war, their weekly rations were:

- 1 ounce (28 grams) cheese

- 3 pints (1.5 litres) milk

- 4 ounces (112 grams) bacon

- 6 ounces (168 grams) meat

- 2 ounces (56 grams) candy

- 1 packet dried egg powder

- 8 ounces (224 grams) sugar

- 2 ounces (56 grams) tea

- 2 ounces (56 grams) butter

- 1 egg (when available)

- Fish unrationed (when available)

Can you imagine living on that for a week? I know I can't.

They don't talk much about those times, the war or their first years here, but the one thing they do say is how hard the transition was. For quite a while, they survived because people they barely knew helped them. It instilled a kindness in them that has filtered down to all of us. I remember one instance as being emblematic of their feelings. We had been camping at Buffalo Pound Lake one weekend. (My parents are ardent campers, having had one trailer or another since I was young. Their most recent jaunt was to Yellowknife and back—at ages eighty-three and seventy-seven!) A nice young couple in a tent was located at the campsite next to us. After two rainy, awful days, the pair was soaked and miserable. My parents invited them to follow us back into town, fixed them lunch, and offered them the use of the shower before sending them on their way. When the couple asked what they could do to repay them, my parents said, "Don't repay us. Pass the kindness along to someone else." To this day, this principle has guided my parents and, through their teachings, us, their children.

My father worked for the phone company for thirty-five years and was a staunch bargainer for the union before taking early retirement. Many of the benefits the Sask-Tel employees enjoyed came from my father's work. My mother worked in the home, taking care of all of us. For years, she volunteered at my elementary school in the library, helping kids with their reading. After several years, the school board named the library in her honour.

As equal partners, my parents raised four children: Susan, Linda, Jennifer, and me. When I was born, Sue was sixteen, Linda was ten, and Jennifer was eight. In fact, my sisters took great glee in telling me that, nine months before I was born, they were on a trip to the mountains, and it was very cold. When I was born, my mother, after three girls, looked at the doctor when he told her it was a boy and cracked, "Are you sure?"

My first concrete memory is the day Sue married for the first time. I was three. While I somewhat remember the sailor suit I wore (more from the pictures than anything else), I vividly remember the car I rode in while going back to the house for the reception in our backyard. The red, quilted, vinyl panels inside the back door are forever etched in my memory.

I guess it was a fairly normal childhood. There are patches of memory after that—my grade one teacher always dressed in a clown outfit for Halloween, I was made to redo a map colouring exercise because my colours were too sloppy and spilled out of the provincial borders.

I remember my father travelling a lot. I think it was mostly union business. He always returned with Dinky or Matchbox toys, mostly space vehicles of some kind. From an early age, I was deeply into science fiction of one form or another. I was three when *Star Trek* was on the first time, and I recall my parents being certain the image of one of the aliens in the closing credits would terrify me. It was my sisters' responsibility to distract me to prevent the supposedly inevitable hysterics. When I finally saw it, unsurprisingly, I had no idea what the fuss was about.

There were always books in the house. Saturday was the day for the library. As soon as I was old enough, I had a library card that was typed in red in order to set it apart from the adult cards, which were typed in black. While my parents were upstairs, I was in the children's section, poring over Dr. Seuss before graduating to Edgar Rice Burroughs and up. It was always something fanciful that would whisk me away to something far beyond what I knew.

I built with Lego, keeping it all in a battered, green tackle box by the TV in the living room. I played with Hot Wheels and Dinky toys, sometimes lining them up in perfect rows around the edges of the living room rug. Before I was ten, you could point at a car on the road, and I could tell you the make and model.

For some strange reason I still can't fathom, though my family loves to embarrass me with the story in front of my friends, I couldn't stand to have "Happy Birthday" sung to me. Most birthdays found me with my hands over my ears, howling "Don't sing!" I must ask my shrink about that someday.

As I grew up, I became more of a loner. My father tells me there were weekends when I would disappear into my room and appear only for meals. I lost myself in comics and building spaceships out of stray model parts and plastic. I wanted to escape more and more because, as I grew up, I strayed farther into the land of the uncool.

The years approaching and into adolescence were hard. I was overweight until the middle of high school. Because kids are brutal, I suffered for it. Even when my weight dropped, I was abused more because I read science-fiction magazines and sucked at sports. Also, like so many of my peers, I knew early (if you'll forgive the cliché) I just wasn't like the other boys. I identified far more with Jaime Summers than Steve Austin. I read Wonder Woman and Black Canary. I thought Storm and Phoenix were infinitely cooler than any of the other X-Men. I just didn't want to sleep with them. In the late seventies in Saskatchewan, I learned early that gay was just about the worst thing you could be.

I once found a gay erotic magazine at a local corner store. I have no idea how it got there because I can't think of anyone who would have openly purchased such a thing in Moose Jaw. I ended up stealing it and poring over it, not really understanding why it appealed to me. There was no hardcore content. The most sexual thing in it was two naked men beside each other, one with an arm slung casually around the shoulder of the other. While looking at those pictures, an understanding of who I was began emerging. Eventually, racked with guilt, I burned it.

As things became clearer, I deliberately set out to lose my virginity. One day, when I was fifteen, I was in the magazine and bookshop where I always bought my comics. At the magazine rack, near the titty magazines, I saw a man reading a magazine like the one I had stolen a year or so before. I made eye contact and held it. When he left the store, I followed him. We chatted and then drove out into the country. On a deserted road, I reached my goal. For the next five years, I rode a roller coaster from thinking I would grow out of it ("It's just a phase") to self-hate ("I'll never do it again"). Needless to say, by leading a double life, I did learn how to lie and cover my tracks early on.

I made the remaining years of high school bearable by finding my way into the drama club. I appeared in nearly every play produced between grade ten and graduation. I gained a certain amount of status for bringing honour to the school. In those moments when the curtain was raised in the gym, I found something that offset the torment. More than that, I found something I was good at that gave me a circle of friends and kept some of the loneliness at bay.

In grade twelve, writing became a part of my life in a creative writing class, a special, limited enrolment class taught by one of the school's English teachers, a noted Saskatchewan poet. All of us had to "audition" to participate. That class offered one of those magic sets of circumstances when lightning strikes. We were an odd mix of students who probably would never have come together in any other situation—the cheerleader, the football player, the Mormon, the Apostolic Christians, the oddballs, the good girl, and the closeted gay teen. All of us left that class with a strange new awareness of our shared gift along with an understanding that these students, who we might have never spent time with, were human as well. In fact, the three people from high school who I remain in contact with were in that class.

In the fall of 1981, I moved to Saskatoon to live with my sister, Linda, and her husband. I began attending the university to earn a bachelor's degree in drama. In many ways, it was quite a growth period. I began coming into my own during those years, meeting people who would shape my life and beginning several of the friendships that would follow me for the rest of my life. Most importantly and, thoroughly anticlimactically, I came out. After years of the internal raging battle, I looked at myself one day and realized it wasn't going away. I told all of my friends and was received warmly and with open arms. However, I did not tell anyone in my family until many years later. To this day, I don't really know why I waited so long. I do remember being thoroughly traumatized at the thought that one or more members of my family might cut me off. It's funny because we're not a demonstrative family (we have too much of the stiff upper lip British reserve for that), but the bonds still run deep. The thought of being cut off from them (as I had seen with so many others) was unbearable. In retrospect, I shouldn't have worried. When Anita Bryant was on her antihomosexual rampage in Florida during the late seventies, I remember hearing a report on the news about her during dinner. (The TV remained on, set to the news, so we could hear it in the other room.) I remember my father saying she should leave people alone and it was no one else's business.

Once I settled the identity issue and following a crazy summer of late nights with my new friends, Diana and Sharon, I moved on to my second year. As the Christmas break was about to begin, I met Gordon Portman. Falling deeply for each other, we had a crazy four-month fling with a dramatic breakup and a reconciliation brought on by a sappy song. When the school year ended, he left for school in Edmonton. We corresponded until he wrote a letter to me, bragging about how happy he was because all of his fellow students thought he was straight. In a fit of drama, feeling this betrayed everything we had meant to each other in that short time, I wrote him a poem, a caustic, breakup haiku. For months, we did not have any contact with each other. Then, one night I was with friends in Saskatoon's only gay bar. Standing near the door, I looked up, and he was there. Taking one look at me, he shouted, "I knew, if I came down here, you would be here!" We've been best friends ever since. Over the years, we've both been sure that we were meant for each other, but never at the same time. Despite the shit we've put each other through, we've always been committed to staying friends. That has held us together so we could finally lay the ghosts of our former romance to rest. As you'll see later, I've been incredibly glad of his friendship.

I learned a lot in my university years…and not just about academics. To this day, I still think of my life actually beginning in those years. I explored myself and the limits of the world around me. I became stronger and more at ease with my sexuality. I fell in love many times and had my heart broken often, but I learned a lot. I acted in many shows throughout those years and made many friends. Some have stayed through the years; some haven't.

In my fourth year, I was lucky enough to be cast in a professional production, the Canadian premiere of *Noises Off* by Michael Frayn. The director said he gave me the role because of my glasses, but that didn't matter. It was an amazing experience as I did a breakneck, physical farce with a group of seasoned, professional actors. That show challenged me in incredible ways, and I think I actually rose to the challenge. Unfortunately, the show led to bad politics and issues with one of my professors. By the time the show ended, I was behind in most of my classes. I made the decision to drop some, just to get to the end of the year. With a bad taste in my mouth about the department, I decided to take time off and work. To this day, I still harbour regret that I didn't finish my degree. However, my path has led me to the person I am today, and I'm quite fond of that person. Once life is on the page, it can't be rewritten. Life is one big final draft.

Once school was over, I got my first job. In the time-honoured tradition of actors everywhere, I waited tables. The financial freedom allowed me to get my first apartment (a tiny bachelor suite with beige walls and hideous orange, brown, and yellow hi-lo carpet) and travel a little. I discovered I was an excellent waiter, and I enjoyed it. I began writing to provide a creative outlet. I wrote science fiction novels (three to date) I tried desperately to sell, thus beginning a thick file of rejection letters.

My process of growing up continued. I had the misfortune of being gay-bashed one night after work. Luckily, I was not badly hurt, but it had a profound effect on my personality. Before, I had often experienced slurs and verbal abuse while I was in public. Being me, I took it all to heart. I often sat in the depths of despair, wondering what I had done to deserve such venom. After I was attacked, something changed. At the first opportunity, I walked home along the same route at the same time of night. I chose not to be afraid because, if I didn't, the bastard that beat me up would have won. I was determined that he not win. After that, the verbal abuse stopped. My theory is that I stopped being a victim after that night. By refusing to knuckle under, I turned a corner and developed some personality traits that (let me tell you) came in handy.

I came out to my family in short bursts. Each and every one of them accepted me without any reservations. I continued writing and moved through a succession of restaurants. I moved into the apartment where I think I was happiest: a rambling, three-bedroom flat in an old building called the McKim. There were pocket doors between the living room and dining room. The floors were hardwood. I also had a beautiful (if nonfunctional) fireplace with emerald green tiles and copper metalwork. I shared the huge place with a succession of roommates. My friend Kim lived upstairs. My friends Travis and Jen lived on the other side of the building. Pauline lived there as well. We often wandered back and forth to and from each other's places or sat together on the communal balconies, sharing a sense of community. To this day, I miss my "family of choice."

If there was a stain on those years, a *bête noire* that plagued me, it was a borderline, compulsive attitude toward sex. Then, I didn't really have many meaningful romantic relationships. Like so many other people, I desperately craved that kind of relationship, but I wanted it too much and often pushed too hard. Aries, don't you know. The desire to find someone else to complete me often led me to use sex to ease loneliness, substituting false intimacy for the real thing. While I was careful, I was also damned lucky. The compulsive behaviours and the survivor's guilt of watching peers and friends die have taken a long time to put in their place.

A big part of my healing happened when my journey through the restaurants of Saskatoon finally led me to a place called Café Browse. Conceived as a café and bookstore combination, it was the first openly gay business in Saskatoon. It was a joy working there. I met so many people, both friends and intimates. When there was a change in ownership, I took on more responsibility, becoming the de facto assistant manager. I became more involved in the bookstore side of things, including ordering titles, maintaining the database, and organizing special events. My lifelong love of books largely reignited during this time, leaving me a little unsatisfied to be serving coffee and lunch.

During my fourth year at the Browse, I met the person who would change everything, leading me away from the prairies and onto the field where the coming battle would be waged.

Early in my illness, my friend Rosie sent me an e-mail. It was one of those chain missives that glorifies friendship. I can always count on her for them. Though I tut-tut the entire concept, I always read them when they arrive. Whoever wrote this particular message divided people into three categories: those in your life for a reason, a season, or a lifetime. According to the theory, all the people in your life belong to one of these categories.

Those in your life for a reason are there for a specific purpose, to teach you something, learn something from you, or effect change in some way. Once the purpose has been accomplished, the person passes from your life.

Some people are in your life for a season. They enter your life and you walk side by side for a period. However, when the time passes, so do they. My friend Brian was like that. We had an intense, passionate friendship for a few years, sharing our exploits and a lot of laughter. We helped each other over breakups. For a while, I was hopelessly in love with him. By the time I was over him, he had fallen in love with someone else. Shortly after that, I met the man I left Saskatoon for. Brian and I spent less time together, and the friendship faded.

Finally, there are those people in your life that stay by your side forever. For me, they are Gordon and Sandra Sprecker, whom I met shortly after meeting Gordon. I had spoken to her once in passing when I saw her wearing an Avengers T-shirt. (I've always been a huge Mrs. Peel fan.) One day, she was painting scenery for *Guys and Dolls*. I was in a pissy mood over some stupid tiff with Gordon, so I bitched at her, carefully avoiding pronouns. We discovered a mutual love of movies and science fiction, and things just went from there. Though we haven't lived in the same city for years, she is still one of my dearest friends. In recent years, she has been struggling to deal with a brain injury (something called a chemical insult), but we still talk regularly. She is happy and settled with a man who takes good care of her.

The first time I met Kerry, the man who changed my life when we fell in love, was in the company of a friend of his, a young pup I was hot for in that doomed, one-sided, "not a chance in hell" sort of way. He was part of a group that was at the bar one night, and I was introduced to him as one of many.

The next time Kerry and I crossed paths, I was setting up the outdoor tables at Café Browse on a sunny summer morning. He came across the street in his suit. I asked where he had been. He said, "To court." Not knowing he was a lawyer, I asked, "Oh, what did you do?" Dead serious, he said he had filed a motion or some such lawyer-type thing, completely missing my meaning. After some polite chitchat, we went our separate ways. We crossed paths a couple of times after that, but it wasn't until a party that our interaction increased.

It was a twenties, forties, or sixties party where you had to dress up in clothing from one of those decades. I was in a thirty-year-old tuxedo that I had just come to possess. At one point in the evening, a pink feather boa was around my neck. Several of my other friends were there, including Kerry. As the evening wore on, he chatted with my friend, Jen, who was in law school a year after him. They swapped horror stories about professors and such. He proceeded to get a little drunk as the evening progressed.

Coincidentally, both of us were getting over breakups. Though painful, mine hadn't been hugely traumatic, but the drink loosened Kerry's tongue. Some creative, quite amusing bitterness was surfacing. After the party, we went to the bar to sit and talk. Half-jokingly, I said I was only interested in meeting "rebound guy," the man you date temporarily after breaking up with someone else. Very flatly, he said he did not have any interest in anything like that. Anyone interested in him would have to take it seriously. It piqued my curiosity, and we agreed to meet on Canada Day for coffee.

When the holiday morning came, we went for something to drink and took a long walk. For hours, we strolled along residential streets, dodging cankerworms hanging from every tree. We talked…and talked…and talked. I discovered we shared a love for comics, having collected many of the same ones. By the end of the day, we were "seeing each other."

Things moved fast after that (maybe too fast), but it seemed right at the time. He spent most of his time at my place, going home to change for work early in the morning. We crossed paths as we went to work and kissed on the street corner, which was quite a big deal for downtown Saskatoon. He moved his computer in and began teaching me how to use it. By September, we were living together.

That fall, my niece Wendy got married. Kerry came with me and met my family for the first time. He was so nervous that he dressed up very prim and proper. (Wendy and Don wanted things to be as informal as possible). He nearly had a fit when I told him he was the first boyfriend my family would meet. It was a major event in my life, my first long-term, successful partnership. Did my gonads do backflips when he was near? No.

All of my life, I've never felt I belonged anywhere. I've spent nearly forty years on this planet wondering when the mother ship would find me and return me to my kind, that is, when I would see myself reflected in someone else's eyes. Before

Kerry came along, I had felt passion that singed my toes. However, the old expression warns, "The flame that burns twice as bright burns half as long." With Kerry, I felt the closest thing to the sense of belonging I yearned for. We were together nearly two years when the move to Toronto came up. I knew he was unhappy in his job. He had switched firms since we had been together and was not any happier with the new one. The job in Toronto seemed like the answer to his prayers. After a great deal of soul-searching, we decided to move.

Unfortunately, the job in Toronto did not bring any measure of satisfaction for him. While struggling with all of the adjustments and his growing discontent, the cracks began showing and growing deeper with each passing day. I began realizing that Kerry's unhappiness was something that came from within. Deep down, he was not satisfied with life or himself. As he needed more from me, I reacted badly and pulled back. I've been a fairly positive person in my adult years, basically quite happy and comfortable in my own skin. In my limited understanding, I could not grasp why he just did not choose to be happier. I now see he was suffering from depression. At the time, I'm afraid I wasn't always patient.

You see, I come from stern, British stock. "Be strong…Pull yourself up by the bootstraps…Get on with life when things don't go your way! Add to that the fact that, if you start making demands of me, I'm just as likely to say no just because I feel pushed. (Aries again.)

So, two people were unsatisfied people without the skills to communicate with each other in times of conflict. (This is another product of my upbringing. We rarely talk about deep subjects in my family, and we tend to just go icy when faced with conflict.) It was only a matter of time.

"It takes two to make a relationship and two to break it," my friend Brian always said. I didn't know how to deal with the conflict, and Kerry was just so deeply unhappy with himself. He needed me to reassure him that he was desirable and worthwhile. I couldn't do it enough. The more he needed, the more I resisted.

When he asked me to move out, though, I felt my world had collapsed. Despite all of the problems, I honestly thought I was going to be in that relationship for the rest of my life. I debated moving home, but I decided to stay because I liked my job. Hope sprang eternal.

Gordon's boyfriend, David, had a spare room in the house he was living in. Because the leaseholder was in Germany, I lived rent-free for the first month. When the leaseholder moved out and transferred the lease to David, I took over a third.

David saved my life that fall. I had a safe, loving home in a strange city I had barely begun to know. I went to work, came home, and worked with my computer to learn more about its ins and outs. I finished my third novel, even though it needed large amounts of work. Surprisingly, I found I had a home here that was independent of Kerry. One of the main things I feared before moving was that I couldn't make a life for myself anywhere besides Saskatoon. But, here I was. I had my own life and the beginnings of my own relationships. It wasn't an easy time, but I actually began feeling like I lived here.

After six months of living apart, just as we were planning to move into the new apartment with an old friend from Saskatoon, Pauline de Jong, I again asked Kerry (in one of those conversations that make you feel like you've been kicked in the gut) if he wanted to be with me. Like every other time, he said, "I don't know." I heard myself saying that wasn't good enough. In that moment, I definitely knew that him wanting to be with me was something we had to start from, not something we had to get to. So we ended, at least romantically.

The subsequent months of cohabitation were brutally hard, growing harder after my diagnosis. It was important to me to try developing a friendship with Kerry, and it took a lot of work. The work became harder when he began a new relationship. The things I wanted for us, he found with someone else.

I don't know if he's in my life for a lifetime, but he's definitely been there for a reason. Like no one else, he opened doors for me. If not for him, I wouldn't be using a computer to write this. If not for him, I would have probably never left Saskatoon. If not for him, I wouldn't have been in Toronto, near the best specialists for my illness. I quit smoking for him. Moreover, he opened the door to the first doctor who recognized that something was seriously wrong.

Three
The Magical Medical Tour

Looking at the title of this chapter, at the joke I often made to all who would listen, it now seems glib and facile. It is a hollow jest that can't begin encompassing the eventual pain and grief, the vomit and blood. However, it's one of the things the Kings (including myself) do. To defuse the power things have to wound us, we laugh at them. Even at my lowest point, after the disease beat and bruised me and I was unsure of where to find hope, I still laughed.

When the tour began on December 16, 1999, Pauline had gone to England for school for eight months. We had sublet her room to James, a (very) young Ryerson student. Kerry and I often joked we didn't get a roommate. We had adopted instead.

On that winter day, I met Dr. Peter Satok for the first time. Peter is one of those unaffectedly handsome men who is unaware of his own looks. With a lovely wife and two beautiful children, he is one of those perfect, picket fence people who we perpetual outsiders always wanted to be. You want to hate him for being so damn perfect, but you can't because he's so genuinely nice. His caring and compassion are absolutely sincere. You never doubt for a second his total commitment to your recovery. There's something straight and true about him, like a landmark or a star to set your course by.

In addition to my need for a checkup and my concerns over my knee, I was concerned about something else. When visiting my home in Saskatchewan, my compulsions resurfaced, and I had skirted the boundaries of safe sex. I was concerned about the risk of HIV infection. At the outset of my first meeting with Peter, I said I wanted to be tested. Taking it all in stride, before I knew it, we were discussing rimming. I thought, "What does a nice straight guy like you know about stuff like this?"

When the cancer diagnosis came, Peter became my touchstone. Though he wasn't the one treating me, I ran everything by him. To keep him informed, I often went straight from one of my treatments to his office. He always gave me brutally frank information as well as honest hope. I always knew I could count on him to cut through all of the double-talk and get at the essence. When it was bad, he just looked at me and, very matter-of-factly, said, "It's bad." Yet, on one of the days I was in his office ranting about my fears and grief, he said he had a huge knot in his stomach at that moment. I was honestly surprised. He always dealt with me in such a reserved fashion, so it seemed unusual this could provoke such a visceral reaction in him. With my tongue getting the better of me, I could only ask, "Why?" It was his turn to seem surprised. He responded, "How could I not feel it?"

When we began, his manner was always textbook "doctor." He was never cold, but expressions of affection were nothing more overt than a firm handshake hello or good-bye. He's been so firmly in my corner that I find myself wanting to give him a hug. I know it isn't right; it would just make him uncomfortable and break that perfect balance of compassion and detachment. Our relationship has changed over the last three years. It has loosened and softened. At that moment, as I so often do, I pushed through that wall and hugged him. The second time, he hugged me back, but it has never happened again.

The relationship you have with a doctor is unique in its contradictions. It is an intimacy like no other. Your doctor sees inside you, sometimes literally. He or she knows your body in a way you can't, a way even your lovers can't. You tell things to your doctor that you tell no one else. I often feel it should be love. Yet, the doctor must remain distant and objective, especially if the doctor is in some way responsible for trying to keep you alive. To struggle against your illness and then watch you die, indulging in love would surely destroy the strongest soul. So, the doctor must care, yet keep himself apart in order to shield himself from caring too much. I don't think our language carries a word that describes that bond between doctor and patient. Perhaps someone should create one.

In that first appointment, after all the poking and prodding (nothing breaks the ice with someone you just met than having his finger up your butt) Peter looked at me and said, "I'm concerned about that mole on your chest. I'm referring you to a dermatologist. And that knee looks terrible. I'm sending you to the sports medicine clinic at Mount Sinai Hospital."

At the time, the waiting list to see a knee specialist in Ontario was six months. Peter knew, if he sent me to the sports clinic, there was a good chance of going over that waiting list. He was right. I have never stopped being grateful for being delivered into Peter's hands.

On January 10, 2000, I found myself at Mount Sinai Hospital on the eleventh floor (a floor I would come to know intimately later) for an appointment with Dr. Ron Taylor. The waiting room for the clinic is also the waiting room for physiotherapy patients. Coming around a corner from the elevators, you reach a reception desk, like an island, standing between the waiting area and you. After going through the processing, I waited and was ushered to a room with several beds separated by candy mint pastel striped curtains. A physiotherapist came and asked questions about my history and watched me walk to measure the difference between my knees. She poked and prodded before leaving me there in my underwear to wait for the doctor.

To this day, Dr. Taylor is a cipher. When he arrived, I listened as the physiotherapist related all of my history to him. He took it in, standing snowy-haired and gruff. I think he probed for a moment or two and gave me the pass I had come for, a referral to Dr. Erin Boynton. He said outright that Peter had known the right way to go about it by sending me to the clinic. He knew full well his cameo role in the drama. He came onstage, delivered his lines with perfection, and exited stage left.

The next day, I had my first appointment with the dermatologist. He looked at the mole and didn't think it was anything serious, but I had to make an appointment for removal and biopsy.

The following week, I went in for a hepatitis vaccination. Because Peter was away, another doctor administered the shot. Two days later, I was again in the dermatologist's office, having the mole removed. The process was painless, a needle of local anaesthetic, a quick nip, and two or three stitches. My chest didn't begin stinging until I was back at work and the anaesthetic wore off.

I think it was then that, somewhere in my mind, the first warning shot went across my bow. Biopsy equals cancer or at least the possibility of it. But it was just a mole, a tiny one at that. Even if the worst played out, how bad could it be? But the seed was planted, as I wrote in my journal that week:

◆   ◆   ◆

01*17*00

I'm tired of doctors and needles and pain. I can't keep facing this stuff alone. I have a biopsy tomorrow and find out on Wednesday whether my knee requires surgery.

I'm very scared. The thoughts of cancer and surgery buzz in my head and fill me with dread.

I just want to be loved. I just want to be held and told it will be all right because everything just looks bleak right now.

◆   ◆   ◆

The day after the biopsy, I had my knee X-rayed and met Dr. Erin Boynton for the first time. Yet another physiotherapist asked all of the same questions as the previous one, took the same history, and related it all to Dr. Boynton when she arrived.

Dr. Boynton is tall and athletic with short, sandy red hair. I noticed a jewelled racquet pin on her lapel. Sitting in the curtained cubicle, I listened to her talk about her daughter with that familiar "proud mom" tone in her voice. After examining me, she told me that she didn't think it was a knee injury because knees don't swell in that particular way (below the kneecap and on the outside). When she talked to me, she did so in a kind, yet doctor-detached way. In the end, she sent me for my first MRI (magnetic resonance imaging) at Princess Margaret Hospital.

For those who have never been to Toronto, Hospital Row lies on the corner of University and Gerrard. Sitting on the three sides of the T-intersection are Mount Sinai, Princess Margaret, Toronto General, and Sick Children's Hospitals. Princess Margaret is the cancer hospital.

My appointment was for 7:45 AM. When my turn arrived, I was ushered through and told to get into a gown. I had to fill out a form swearing I did not have any metal implanted in my body, had never worked with metal, had never had metal in my eye, and had never welded. It was the exact same questionnaire I completed the previous week for Dr. Boynton. After removing my glasses, watch, and jewellery, I was ushered into the actual room.

An MRI machine basically looks like a huge, room-sized doughnut with an aperture barely large enough for a person to fit into. Blind without my glasses, I was led to the platform and placed on it. My legs were arranged in an optimum position (one painful to maintain). I was given huge earphones to shut out the sound of the machine and slid into the tiny hole. I'm just glad I'm not claustrophobic.

The scans themselves lasted anywhere from three to nine minutes, totalling about thirty to forty minutes. While scanning, the machine's noise is seismic. The cadences of the different scans pound at you with a rhythm you can feel and hear on the floor below. In position, I could only see the timer above my head, counting down the seconds of each scan. I did my best to remain perfectly still, but my mind was numb at the frightening foreign quality of it all. It was eventually over, and I put on clothes and jewellery. I went back to work.

While we waited for answers from the MRI, I went to physiotherapy. I went three times to a clinic in the evenings, seeing a different therapist each time. They manipulated the joint and prescribed exercises. However, in the two weeks until I saw Dr. Boynton again, there was little change. Because they didn't know what was happening inside the joint, they were justifiably reluctant to aggressively treat it.

On the Friday after my first physiotherapy appointment, I had the stitches on my chest from the mole removal taken out. Another doctor performed the procedure because the original one had moved his practice.

When I returned to see Dr. Boynton on February 9, the MRI results were in. I had a "mass" in my knee. Isn't that a lovely, bland expression? If you spend any time around doctors, you will hear plenty of those vague, "I'm not sure, so I'm saying nothing" expressions, carefully neutral to avoid panicking you. When you've been on the treadmill as long as I have, your brain automatically translates them into real, emotionally loaded English words. However, at the time, my doctor-to-English dictionary hadn't formed. I only knew I had a "mass."

A "mass"? Protons have mass. Catholics have Mass. Even in my stunned state, I knew knees weren't supposed to have "mass."

◆   ◆   ◆

02*09*00

…I don't know how people manage to deal with chronic, severe pain. This pain is strong enough that it keeps me from sleeping through the night or ever really being comfortable and it exhausts me most of the time. I feel drained of energy. And there are times I would give anything to have it stop. (If I had only known!)…

…I keep having flashes of having to lose my leg, endure radical chemotherapy, or something. One way or another, I just want this settled.

◆   ◆   ◆

Looking back now, I find I forgot just how bad the pain was on a day-to-day basis. Spurred by this journal entry, I'm beginning to find the memories again. Walking, something that had always been my favourite exercise, was difficult for any length of time. Kerry and I went for a walk one day, just through the neighbourhood, and we had barely gone a few blocks before I was visibly favouring my leg. The ache, though it varied in intensity, was bone deep and ever present, whether the leg was straight or bent. Sitting at the information desk at work processing orders or performing system maintenance on our computer was difficult because I could never get comfortable. It's amazing what the mind forgets. In the last few months of 1999, my mobility deteriorated rapidly. Merely climbing the stairs into my apartment became a Herculean task. The distension in the joint was becoming more obvious.

Having discovered the mass in my knee, Dr. Boynton stamped the pass and passed me along to the next link in the chain, bypassing yet another six-month wait. I met orthopaedic surgeon Dr. Jay Wunder on February 21, after waiting in a hall plastered with posters with graphic photos and information about cancers. My mind resisted the omen, the smoke on the horizon. That didn't mean me. That was what happened to other people. All I had was a "mass."

Eventually, I was ushered into an examination room across the hall from the doctor's office on the fourth floor of the hospital. A resident came in to take my history. This became a habit. At every appointment, a student, resident, or some equivalent took my history and asked the same questions to determine my status or progress.

Once I played "I'll take personal medical information for a thousand, Alex," I waited for the doctor. Waiting is another thing you get used to. It's no one's fault. There are just lots of people in line with complicated problems and illnesses that require time to deal with. Cancer doesn't keep a schedule.

Jay Wunder is a tall, lean man with a slight stoop to his shoulders, the posture tall people sometimes develop as if they're trying not to be tall. Dr. Wunder initially gives an impression of youth, but subtle flecks of grey are in his hair. Later, in conversations with various people, I would learn he was perhaps the best man in the city, perhaps the country, to be treating my illness.

After a discussion of history and symptoms, he felt around the joint and discussed the precise angle of insertion for the biopsy needle with the resident. With a gentle smile and firm handshake, he left. The resident arranged me on the table, another uncomfortable position. He gave me two separate needles of local anaesthetic. Why is it that they can give you something to make you not hurt, but it always hurts? Once the anaesthetic took effect, he took a needle that looms in my memory as having the bore of a ballpoint pen and inserted it into my knee.

This was not like the last biopsy, no innocent snip and couple of stitches. Initially, there was not any pain, just the sensations of something unfamiliar probing deep inside the joint, a place where nothing but your own tissues should be. As the resident took samples, I felt a pinching sensation as he plucked pieces of the mass. I forget the exact number of samples he took, but it was at least five or six. One of the last ones must have hit a nerve because a sudden jolt of searing pain shot through my leg. I jerked so hard that I'm surprised I didn't break the needle off inside my knee. When the pain ebbed, we finished up. He showed me the vial with the innocent-looking pink bits of flesh floating in it.

And there was blood. Great scarlet smears of it stained the drapes over the bed as well as my leg. After cleaning up, he put a small bandage over the tiny entry wound, but the blood seeped through the bandage before I had even left the room. By the time I reached work, there were two tiny, brown stains on the fabric of my pants.

Four
Cusp

After the biopsy, I waited for a week. I don't remember being frightened, but I don't know if I was handling it well or if I was in complete denial.

In my early twenties, I was in a car accident. While riding in the passenger seat of a minivan, we were broadsided by a truck. The minivan flipped over and was sent into the back end of a parked car. I remember seeing the truck coming at us and having just enough time to register the inevitable collision. In that moment, as time slowed to a crawl, I don't remember feeling fear, just a sort of calm realization that I could only wait to see how it turned out and how bad the damage would be. "Well, there's nothing I can do about this now, so I guess I'll just hold on and see how it turns out." Like that feeling that came over me in those last seconds before the collision, I knew I could only hang on. I went to work, watched TV, checked e-mail, and did all of the normal things that were my life at the time. I had been keeping my out-of-town circle informed; however, all of it was in a glib, jaunty, depthless tone. I was utterly denying what I felt.

The following Tuesday (the leap day of the leap year) came. I reported to the twelfth floor of Mount Sinai. (Every visit, I saw Dr. Wunder in a different place.) This hallway was also filled with posters about cancer and people with cancer waiting for chemotherapy. I sat alone and waited, feeling stirrings of dread. This was where the cancer patients were. This is where I was. Was that significant? There was nothing to do except wait.

After a time, I was ushered into yet another pastel cubicle to wait some more with only out-of-date magazines for company. I heard Dr. Wunder a few cubicles over, talking to another young man about some problem with his leg. (The details are now lost in the haze of that afternoon.) I heard him leave the other cubicle and tell his resident-of-the-day that he now had to tell a man he had a synovial sarcoma in his knee.

And then he came through my door.

I played dumb, stunned by what I had heard. He went through it all, saying he had thought it was something called a PVNS, but the pathology confirmed the sarcoma. He asked if I had any questions, but I couldn't think of any in my dazed state. He said I should write any that came to mind later so I would remember them. He said I needed to talk to his secretary, Dave, about making an appointment for a CT scan of my lungs. If tumour cells had broken from the primary site and travelled elsewhere in my body (a process called metastasis), they would have lodged in the natural filter of the lungs. He said there would be more pathology sessions and I should call for another appointment as soon as the CT was scheduled. Then, putting his hand on my shoulder, he said they would take good care of me.

I stumbled through my talk with Dave as we arranged the necessary appointments. I then left the hospital and began slowly walking back to work. I had left early, and they didn't expect me back. I thought about what I knew about cancer as I walked, losing myself in the safe, repetitive motion that did not require any conscious effort. The only thing I knew about cancer was that Sandra's father had it and he had died. I remembered the sight of her on the day of his funeral, standing hand in hand with her mother, sister, and brother on that windy day at the cemetery. I remember her weeping in my arms afterwards. That was the extent of my knowledge: cancer equals death.

I was drawn back to the mall. My world was suddenly insane, and the store and staff provided a safe zone, just like they had been when Kerry and I split up. I took refuge in my responsibilities. In that haze, I needed to see Margot to tell her what was happening. We were going to have to work things out, including my schedule, the staff, and the operation of the store. She was on the phone when I came in. She looked up at me, and I mouthed, "It's bad." She hung up, and I told her what I knew. She knew what I was going through. Several years before, she had cancer surgery performed on her jaw at the same hospital. Once that was through, I went home and began phoning the people I loved.

◆   ◆   ◆

03*01*00

I have cancer.

Three little words, innocuous ones yet loaded like the barrel of a howitzer. So much of our lives turn on these three-word phrases. "I love you." "Let me help."

I have cancer.

The lump in my knee is malignant. We are waiting for new pathology reports, but it seems to be looking bad. Dr. Wunder, who, by all reports, is the leading man in this field in the city, if not the country, tells me that, if detected early, the cure rate is 95 percent. There will be surgery and radiation.

Peter, my general practitioner, tells me the treatment for this is aggressive. The surgery will remove the sarcoma and, depending on the incursion, bone as well. This is not going to be pretty or easy.

I have to go for a CT scan of my lungs because that's where it has gone if it has spread. Dr. Wunder says he doesn't think this has happened.

I panic at the slightest stitch in my side or shortness of breath.

I think I'm handling it all as best I can—that is, the shock and denial.

It nearly killed me to tell my parents. Dad took it on the chin. Mum cried and had to hang up. She tried though. She listened to it all before it got to her. (The next time we talked, she apologized for losing control. I was stunned. Like anyone is unreasonable to lose control in the midst of this.)

I can't begin to describe how weird this feels. Everything seems perfectly normal one minute. Then it all seems like this spectacularly hideous joke, like a Twilight Zone episode.

◆   ◆   ◆

I called my closest friends and my sister Linda. By then, I was choking on the words. I asked her to tell Sue. I asked my parents to tell Jennifer. At the first opportunity to just sit and stop a moment, I cried huge, gut-shaking sobs that left me feeling like I had been mugged.

When I talked to Sandra, she said something I took to heart. She told me that, however I thought I was going to react, I needed to throw it all out. There were no rules. During the same conversation, the phrase that became my mantra and the title of this book came to light. She said, "All you have to do is breathe." When all of this became too intense and overwhelming, breathing was the only thing I had to accomplish. Everything else could be postponed.

I veered through every possible emotional state in those initial days. In some moments, I felt almost calm, a sense there was little I could do. Linda expressed it as a feeling that was now up to the professionals to deal with. I only had to follow orders.

"Be here at this time for this procedure." Okay.

"This is the time for your CT scan." Okay.

"We're sending you for a course of radiation." Okay.

It was my place to do as I was told. On other days, I was close to insane.

◆   ◆   ◆

I don't know if I can do this. I don't know if I can face this coming storm of pain and fear and world-shaking change.

I feel so alone, which sounds odd even to my ears. I have this amazing bedrock of love from my friends and family, yet there's this time lag. Everyone is so far away. Kerry tries, but, as always, he is caught up in his own life. He's gone out tonight. On some level, I wanted him to stay, but I know I don't just want him. I need some other caregivers. I can't deal with it all coming from him.

A flood of tears came—anguish, fear, doubt—wracking my body and heart. It passed. I'm back trying to maintain the positivity I'm going to need to see me through this.

Just breathe…

◆   ◆   ◆

My CT scan was scheduled for March 7 at 9:00 AM. That same afternoon, I was scheduled for my next appointment with Dr. Wunder. I then scheduled an appointment with Dr. Satok for 5:30 to touch base and keep him informed. The Magical Medical Tour played on.

The Saturday after my diagnosis, I found myself alone in the house. Kerry was off somewhere. I went down to Queen Street West to shop. I wandered around for a couple of hours in a daze. I stopped at the Silver Snail to check out the comics and action figures. I went to the local Chapters, where I found a journal.

I had decided to get something more special than the plain, black books I usually wrote in. I wanted something special to record the memories of the coming months. On the racks, I found a coil-bound, blank book from the Metropolitan Museum of Art. It was sepia with a sixteenth-century pen sketch of an angel on the cover. It seemed like a good omen.

On the first page, before writing another word, I wrote my mantra, framing it with a Nick Bantock postcard. As time passed, I filled the book with thoughts and the accounts that became this book. I inserted photos, business cards of my various doctors, and appointment cards. I copied the quotes that spoke to me, carefully inscribing them from the book I have been compiling for years. I kept it with me wherever I went, writing in it whenever the thoughts came to me.

When the day of my CT scan arrived, I showed up early with plenty of time. (I'm always early. I get the sweats if I show up late for anything. I'd rather be twenty minutes early than five minutes late.) The fifth floor of Mount Sinai houses the medical imaging department. It was left of the elevators in a hallway painted in another of those sickening pastel shades found nowhere else except hospitals. I presented my hospital card. (I had two now to prove my patient status wherever I went: one for Mount Sinai and one for Princess Margaret.) I took a seat in the waiting room. When my turn arrived, I went through the door to a set of dressing rooms where I took off my shirt and put on another shapeless hospital robe. I was ushered into a cold, stark, white room, like something from a dystopian vision of the future, with another giant, ominous-looking machine. It looked somewhat like the MRI machine, but it was smaller. A bench raises you into the aperture. Above you, a blood red laser guide warns against looking directly into the beam.

The technicians arranged me on the table and disappeared into their shielded compartment to protect them from whatever radiations I was going to be exposed to. There were breathing instructions "Breathe in…Breathe out…Breathe in and hold your breath." I heard the machine buzz, but it was not nearly as clamorous as the MRI. I then heard a disembodied voice from the control bunker say, "Nice necklace, Stephen."

It was the silver ankh I wear around my neck. Its chain hung just low enough to glow white hot in the scan's image. The nice woman came in, pulled it out of the way, and, with a chuckle, continued. It was over quickly, and I left.

I must have done something in the intervening hours before I saw Dr. Wunder at 1:00, but I don't remember. The time is blank. Even if I had to wait for the scan, I can't account for a couple hours. I know, when I went for the CT appointment, Kerry wasn't with me. However, when I went to see Dr. Wunder, he was. But I can't account for the intervening time or how we got together.

My appointment was at the fracture clinic on the fifth floor where Dr. Wunder was seeing patients that afternoon. There was another wait and yet another curtained cubicle. While I waited, I heard Dr. Wunder talking to a woman in the next cubicle. There was nothing except a curtain separating us, so, despite not wanting to eavesdrop, I heard everything. The woman had a tumour in her arm that had broken a bone as it grew. As I listened, the doctor had to say her cancer had metastasized to her lungs and her condition was serious. When Dr. Wunder left her to make arrangements before coming to me, I waited and listened to her cry.

When Dr. Wunder came in to see me, two physiotherapy students from the University of Toronto accompanied him. There is nothing like sitting in front of complete strangers in your underwear.

The second round of pathology confirmed the diagnosis. There was not a great surprise. Dr. Wunder drew lines on my knee to show where the sarcoma was. My heart skipped a beat. It was large, having completely infiltrated the joint. I would go for radiation treatment and then have surgery to remove the joint and replace it with an artificial one. He explained, when removing a tumour like this, a two-centimetre margin of healthy tissue had to be around it to ensure complete removal. He thought he might be able to save the kneecap and the patellar ligaments along the joint's inside edge, which would increase the mobility I would regain afterward. Because the tumour is close to the skin, they planned to remove the muscle, take a flap from the muscle below the knee, reattach it above the joint, and complete a skin graft over it. My fears about surgery were coming true with a vengeance. Recovery was going to be a long, hard journey. It would take a long time and a lot of work, but, at the time, perhaps due to shock and denial, I felt it was a fight I could win. I think I just took it all in, shifting into kick-ass mode. I did my best to absorb it while, not completely, pushing grief and fear down.

At one point, I was sitting in a chair, and Dr. Wunder was on a short stool at my feet. I was sitting in my underwear. He wore scrubs, and his legs were spread. My foot was resting against his inner thigh as he filled in the students about my history and diagnosis. While he spoke, he casually reached up to feel the lymph nodes in my groin for lumps. They were clear, but I thought, "Under different circumstances, the position would have been quite pleasant." Even with cancer, I'm a big, old tart.

The most important thing was that the CT showed nothing abnormal in my lungs. Dr. Wunder said I would receive a call once my radiation was arranged. Again, he asked if I had any questions. I had written some down, but he had already provided most of the answers. I promised to write more questions down. We said good-bye again. The earnest students wished me luck, addressing me as Mr. King as they followed Dr. Wunder to the next patient.

I think I must have gone back to work, but it's a blank again. I know I went to see Peter that afternoon, just to fill him in on everything I knew. He said, due to funding cuts by good old Mike Harris, the premier who had decimated Ontario health care, there was a shortage of radiation technicians in Ontario. Instead of setting a precedent of hiring more technicians, cancer patients were being sent to Buffalo, staying in hotels for weeks, and receiving treatments there. Does that sound insane to you, too? Or is it just me?

Looking straight at me in the eye, he said, "If they want to send you to Buffalo, go to Buffalo!" In retrospect, it was one of those clues that things were deadly serious. However, in my addled state, I didn't really pick up on it. Perhaps it's a good thing. Despite the brave face I put on for the world, deep down I was terrified. However, as I have so often done in my life, I refused to let anyone see it.

Five
Radiation

The next day, March 8, I was supposed to be in a major human resources meeting for work. I bailed out and lay on the couch instead, exhausted and overwhelmed. While I stared vacantly at the TV, Dr. Boynton called to see how I was doing.

There were many of those small kindnesses in those days. Dr. Boynton's secretary, Barbara, and Dr. Wunder's secretary, Dave, both made sure I knew I could call if I needed anything. My regional manager and the human resources director both let me know that the company would do everything it could. A manager from another store, who had been through cancer the previous year, came to see me and told me what to expect.

In the many dark moments, it was easy to feel I didn't have much support because I didn't have many close friends in Toronto. But, as I wrote in my cancer journal, huge, warm hands were holding me, and I received great waves of support from all sides. I may not have known these people well. I may not ever be close friends with them, but they all gave something of themselves to make this easier for me.

After the call from Dr. Boynton, Dave phoned from Dr. Wunder's office. My first appointment with the radiation oncologist had been scheduled. I would not have to wait or go to Buffalo. I just had to go to Princess Margaret Hospital the following day.

Much later, I discovered I was treated with radiation and not chemotherapy because soft tissue cancers are not responsive to chemotherapy. Chemo is prescribed in cases in which the cancer has been spread via metastasis. The cancer is hit with chemotherapy to try to deal with all of the affected areas. Because there was no sign of any spreading in my case, radiation was the chosen course of action.

The next morning, I added another doctor to my collection. Dr. Charles Catton, my radiation oncologist, has a somewhat jaunty manner. Jolly is the only word I can think to describe him. After briefing me on the process and providing pamphlets with information on radiation and its side effects, we laughed at a lame joke about the right knee being the wrong knee and the left knee being the right knee. When he laughed, he tossed his head back. His body shook. I always feel good about someone who laughs without restraint. It was interesting to note that he had an English accent, as did his nurse, Susan, and the first technician I saw, Jane. Considering my heritage, I took it as a good omen.

At one point, Dr. Catton said I was an emergency. I felt my stomach lurch. Was this somehow worse than I thought? Could it actually have been worse? I realize that sounds odd. I mean, I had cancer, right? How could I have doubted it was anything except an emergency? I think medical professionals never sound freaked or uncertain. Dr. Wunder only sounded calm and professional. Any emotion or alarm was never in his voice. I found I couldn't help being anything except fairly calm. People who are fearful or upset betray it in their voices and their manner, don't they? This was my first serious illness and my first experience with medical professional detachment. To my thinking, if someone appeared calm and unconcerned, they either didn't give a shit or the situation wasn't that terribly serious. My psyche took the situation and made it smaller and more manageable.

When I asked about being an emergency, Dr. Catton explained there were only two categories of radiation patients: "You can wait," and "Emergency." When he discussed me with Dr. Wunder on his rounds, they decided I needed to be in treatment right away.

As I wisecracked in my journal that night, being declared an emergency was better than being declared a disaster area.

My first step was a trip to the simulator. Similar in setup to a radiation treatment room, but without the functioning equipment, the simulator room is where two technicians determine the optimal position for treatment. I donned a gown and climbed onto the table. The technicians manipulated me and, once the proper position was found, drew guide lines on my leg with a marker. They then permanently tattooed four pinprick marks into my skin. The marker lines would fade and would be redrawn several times over the next five weeks. However, three of those tiny black dots remain. Only one was lost in the surgery.

Once everything was finalized, they took a Polaroid of me to use as a reference. I surprised them by asking them to take another for me. I stuck the photo in my cancer journal. The overexposed image of my torso, pale legs, and work socks with a weight holding down my ankle was labelled, "And so begins the complete loss of my dignity."

With Polaroid and pants in hand and wearing a hospital gown so well worn that the hospital's logo was nearly faded away, I was led down the hall to the actual treatment room. Behind a huge, lead sliding door, I found the room where I would spend the next five weeks and the people with whom I would spend that time.

Shannon, fair and blonde with crystal blue eyes, became the one I was closest to. She had a wicked sense of humour, and something was always conspiratorial about our interactions. It was like we were two naughty children. Jerry was the physical opposite to Shannon. He was Greek with dark skin and jet-black hair. I have always had a weakness for the dark-skinned, Mediterranean type, and I developed a wee crush on our Jerry. It was hopeless, as I knew he was straight. Hey, my knee was messed up, not my libido. Last of the core group was Geri, a little older and sandy-haired with a lovely smile and an easy laugh. (I was making wisecracks, go figure. I was using humour as armour once again.)

Any trepidations I might have had disappeared when I walked through the door and heard Shania Twain on the radio and saw the glow-in-the-dark dinosaurs hanging from the ceiling. I climbed on the table with a smile on my face.

The procedure itself is nothing. Once in position on the bed, they turn off the lights and use laser targeting lights to help them guide you into position. With a remote control three times the size of one for a TV, the bed is lifted into range of the U-shaped machine. Adjustments are made, the beam is focused, and the technicians scatter out of the room to their control computers outside. The machine buzzes for about thirty seconds. It then turns on its axis to shoot at you from beneath and buzzes again. And you're done.

I wrote in my journal that night.

◆   ◆   ◆

03*09*00

...fuck me, this is happening fast!

I feel like I've been shot from a cannon. I only found out about this ten days ago. In those ten days, my world has been turned upside down and sideways.

I wrote in my e-mail newsletter tonight that I feel a combination of wanting to howl in pain and fear, scream in rage, and thank all the gods for my luck all at the same time.

And buried underneath it all is the terrible feeling that no one will ever want me like this. Especially once the disfigurement happens. Which makes it quintuply hard when Kerry spends the night with his new man, like he's doing tonight.

I want to feel good for him. In fact, I'm glad he has some escape from this. But there's no escape for me. This is 24/7 and right now I think I'd trade my soul for someone to hold me in his arms tonight.

◆   ◆   ◆

Those feelings often returned in the coming weeks. In her book, Gilda Radner wrote of how lonely a disease cancer is. I came to know this as my fight went on. I often felt like I was on one side of a glass wall with *them*—the unbroken ones; the healthy of cell—on the other side. For me, there was a strong sense that, if you hadn't been through it, you couldn't possibly understand or grasp the implications. How do you describe it to someone who doesn't know the lingo, the vernacular of cancer or even of life-threatening illness? My own feelings were so jumbled and out of control that I couldn't conceive of trying to explain them when I couldn't even begin to order them myself. How I seethed at Kerry in my mind during those dark days.

◆   ◆   ◆

03*11*00

Kerry's gone out for dinner and nookie with Ken again. And the jealousy rages in me, fuelled by the epic, gothic fear that no man will ever want me again. Even if I met someone tomorrow, what do I say? "So, Stephen, tell me about yourself." "Well, I have cancer." What kind of date would that be? A last one. And once this is all over? There I'll be…with a leg like an Amish quilt. Bit of a turnoff.

Which leaves me here, exhausted and desperate for companionship. No arms to hold me in the night and the deep fear I'll never find that comfort ever again.

◆   ◆   ◆

03*13*00

I am furious at Kerry. After disappearing to his boy toy's house from Saturday 6:00 PM to Sunday 10:30 PM, he's back there again.

So much for the promises of being there through this.

I hope fuck boy is worth it because Kerry's lost a shitload of my esteem and respect. And, I think, my love.

I can't do this alone. And if he can't follow through, I need to find someone to take his place.

Linda and I cried together on the phone tonight. I called her to blubber a bit over my rage and betrayal. She wishes she could be here to hold my hand. I do, too.

But, for now, I just have to be strong.

◆   ◆   ◆

03*15*00

Had it out with Kerry last night. Lots of Scarlett O'Hara histrionics on my part (lots of which was the disease talking). Basically, we are both just winging it. Neither one of us knows how to handle this. We're back on an even keel for now.

◆   ◆   ◆

The one thing this disease did was give Kerry and me the break we needed. We finally realized, even though we had broken up, we were just having an odd, asexual nonrelationship.

With the clarity of hindsight, I now can see he was just trying to rebuild his life after the divorce as I was. He was just at a different stage, but no one ever wants their ex to move on first. He was falling in love again. The layers of resentment at him finding someone first were inextricably fused with my rage and terror at facing my disease.

However, the continuing love and support of my friends, so far in distance, offset the anger and loss. It was still there though, beneath my very skin, buried in a different set of cells than my cancer. My friend Debra wrote this in an e-mail.

◆   ◆   ◆

Stephen,

Your doctors sound wonderful, Stephen. Although I know you must be terrified of all the unknown things that are going on and will go on, I have nothing but confidence and good vibes about the people looking after you and that they know exactly what they are doing.

With all the love and support you have, I hope things will emotionally be somewhat easier, even though none of us can take your radiation treatments for you. You know, if I could take away some of the pain and fear, I would.

I have a thought for you. During your radiation, I want you to think of a beautiful place (a beach perhaps). On this beach are all of your friends and all the people who love you. We are mixing fabulous fruity drinks and listening to the breeze in the trees and the waves on the ocean.

We are all relaxed and laughing sitting around you together, talking about peaceful, humorous, lovely things. The air is warm, and the day is stretching out before us like a gift. The day is perfect. All you feel is love, support, and the sun on your face.

I want you to know how important you are to so many people, Stephen. If love can speed up your treatment, you'll be fine in NO TIME!!!!

Take Care
Talk to you soon
Love,
Debra

◆   ◆   ◆

She wasn't the only one. Every day, after every update I sent, my e-mail was filled with messages of love and support, like sandbags shoring up a barrier against floodwaters. And the days of the treatments passed. It amazes me how the extraordinary becomes ordinary and how the most extreme circumstances can just become part of your routine.

◆   ◆   ◆

03*31*00

There are moments in the fight with cancer, moments of brutal clarity.

Most of the time, life is relentlessly normal. The sun comes up, and people go to their jobs, battling traffic or cramming themselves grumpily onto public transit. Everyone has to earn a living, and most couldn't give a shit about your sarcoma or your treatment. A precious few might, if they were aware. But, in some cases, like mine, there is no outward sign of the rogue cells eating away at your flesh. So they move on unaware.

Then come those moments of vicious insight, like a two-by-four to the head or a bone-crunching body blow.

I have cancer.

And, in less than two months, I will be losing my knee to it.

Suddenly, all else pales and, fades into the background. You just want to scream at everyone you pass, becoming another of the random crazies on a big city street corner.

In the end, you just go on about your business. And another moment passes...and then another. The feeling passes. You just have to worry about getting to work and braving transit.

And life, for you as well, goes on.

◆   ◆   ◆

Every weekday for the next five weeks, I was at Princess Margaret for radiation treatment at some point in the day. On some days, it was in the morning. On some days, it was in the early afternoon. On others, it was at the end of the day. Each appointment was neatly noted in my green appointment card with the bar code sticker on the outside.

Every day I left work, walked down the mall to the subway station, and took the subway that travelled down the loop to Union Station and back north along University Avenue to Queen's Park Station. From there, I walked the half-block to the hospital.

Once inside, I took the glass elevator facing the soaring four-story atrium down to sublevel two. (I love glass elevators. I love the sensation of the world falling away or rising to meet your feet). I swiped my green card through the bar code reader, announcing to the computer and my team of technicians that I was there and ready. From there, I walked down a hall and turned left into the waiting room.

The waiting room was always full. It didn't matter what time of day I was there. People were always in most of the chairs. It was an eye-opener for me. Before, I had barely known anyone who had dealt with or was facing cancer. Suddenly, I was in a room full of people dealing with it. (I later discovered that some of the people had travelled from elsewhere for their treatments because no radiation facilities were where they lived.) I suddenly found myself part of a different population, a subculture of people with cancer. And this population was a large one.

Many of the other patients had someone with them, a loved one, spouse, child, or sibling. You could see familial bonds in their faces. On some days, someone was with me. Once or twice, Kerry came, but I found myself resisting his presence as I felt the pressures of the complex restructuring of our relationship in the face of my illness. In my own perversity, I wanted someone with me—but not him, dammit! On many occasions, I pushed him away and then unfairly blamed him for not being there.

Gordon came with me once, getting the tour of the room and the explanation of the machine and its workings. The technicians were great. Any time someone was with me, they took great pains to explain the procedure and make them as comfortable as they had made me.

On most days, I went alone. I waited each day because I always arrived early. On some days, the unit was on time. On other days, they were behind. On some days, I had something with me to read. On others days, I read the ancient magazines. (One day, I read a Canadian decor magazine that ceased publication twenty years ago.) On some days I just sat, unable to focus on anything.

After the wait, I donned the soft, faded robe and climbed on the table for my treatment. Five minutes later, I was on my way back to work.

This was my life for five weeks. My manager and staff shouldered an extra share of my work for those weeks, never once complaining. They just took it as a routine part of the day. My treatments became a normal part of the running of the store.

Every week, I saw Dr. Catton for a checkup to monitor for side effects. The skin on my knee reddened, and there was some fatigue. However, that was the extent of it. I often stopped to see Peter to communicate and keep him informed. My connection with him was vital to me in those days, keeping me in touch with my reality check. Between the boundaries of my treatment schedule, the emotional roller-coaster ride continued though.

◆   ◆   ◆

03*20*00

Eight treatments down and seventeen more to go. The skin's looking pink, ruddy in colour.

The pain has changed. Before, it felt like a constant pressure, outward or sideways. Now, the feeling is more like a pull, like the feel of a scar that stretches but is tight against the play of muscles.

Peter and Shannon both say it's good. It means the radiation is doing what it's supposed to. Peter says it means the tumour is shrinking. That's good.

Emotionally, it's been a rough day.

It's a bitch being the strongest person I know. I need a rock, someone who can shoulder this for a while so I can fall apart all over them, blubber out some of this pain and fear, and just be held.

There's no one in my life like that. Kerry has a good, kind heart, but he's weak. Gordon and David try, but they both have so much on their plates right now.

I just don't have the strength to direct people right now. Everyone looks to me to call them or tell them what I need. All my energy is so caught up in just trying to get a handle on this. I just want some people to seek me out, to phone once in a while. But the phone doesn't ring.

◆   ◆   ◆

Self-pity is an easy route to take in a situation like mine. As you can see, I wasn't immune to its pull. My phone did ring, but, because I didn't have much of a social life, there were too many moments alone, filled only with silence. This was a very fertile ground for self-pity and fear. Linda called often. So did my parents. I was not alone, yet the seductiveness of feeling like no one knew or understood often took hold of me in those days.

At one point, I called an ex-boyfriend, Kelly. We had a long-distance relationship several years ago that failed when neither one of us was ready to move to be with the other. Our attempt at friendship just petered out, and I had never called after I moved. There didn't seem to be any point. Now, in the desire to bring more people into my corner, I called. I know. It was shameless.

When we spoke, because of the Saskatoon grapevine, he knew I was in Toronto. He just assumed we would run into each other someday. We chatted amiably for a few minutes until he asked how I was. When I hesitated, he asked bluntly, "What's wrong?" When I told him, the first words out of his mouth were "How can I help?" Once again, I saw how cancer could bring out the best in people.

Even at the time, on some level, I knew I was hoping to restart something, that is, to dredge open the past, if only temporarily. As it turns out, he was happily involved with someone new. I remember leaving him the first time we got together and thinking the three men I had significant relationships with were all here in the same city and happily involved in relationships with other people. The only constant in all three situations was me, so the responsibility for the failure of the relationships must lie at my feet. I still wonder about it sometimes, but I now know that most of that feeling was the disease talking.

The disease spoke often, colouring my reactions to everything at some point or another. It often left me so emotionally exhausted and drained that my hands shook. I remember going out one night to have dinner with my friends Carolyn and Paul. On the streetcar, a wave of emotion spread over me. Afterwards, I wrote it was a good thing my illness was not imminently terminal because I would have happily "gone into the light" at that moment. My dead relatives were at the other end of the tunnel, calling my name. If I could have, I would have immediately joined them. However, I was relatively healthy with nothing except some knee pain to mark my illness.

When I discussed the feeling with my friend Kim, who lived in Saskatoon, she raised an interesting point. She said that must make it harder. If you find yourself so terribly ill that there is no hope of recovery and if there is nothing except pain and your quality of life has deteriorated without any hope of recovery, you have the option of letting go. I have never kept this feeling secret. If I ever did find myself in that position, I could easily shuffle off this mortal coil.

Ignoring the disease and refusing treatment would have only led to the pain and degeneration of life that letting go would have released me from. There was no option except continuing to fight and carry on with treatment, regardless of where it led.

If there was any doubt about the King tradition of using humour to deal with difficult situations, this e-mail from my niece definitely laid it to rest.

◆   ◆   ◆

Rooting for you…
Stephen:
I'm sure you're not surprised to learn I've been getting updates on the knee-thing from Mom via Lin, and I suspect you're probably just sick of the whole thing, but I wanted to let you know I'm thinking about you and thought you could use a giggle. So, here you go (and please take this in the spirit in which it was intended):

Top Ten Reasons Why Radiation Treatment and Surgery Could be Good:
10. Lots of downtime to catch up on All My Children.
9. Sympathy from roommates means no dishes for months!
8. You can sit on those reserved seats on buses and streetcars and not feel guilty about it.
7. After surgery, crutches can be used as a weapon in crowds.
6. Four Words: Fun with Geiger Counters!
5. During convalescence, you'll have a cane you can shake at squeegee kids while saying things like, "In my day, we were content to just pierce our ears!"
4. Choose from great nicknames like "Radiation Man" and "Fallout Boy."

3. Excellent chance to scope out single doctors.
2. Head maintains that "just shaved" smoothness with no effort.
1. Radiation machine could malfunction and turn you into a crime-fighting superhero.

Anyways, call or write if you ever feel like it, or just remember, I'm thinking about you.
Lots of love,
Pam

◆   ◆   ◆

04*03*00

Haven't written much because it seems not much of note has gone on—just the day-to-day cancer grind. Every day, I stop what I'm doing at work, get on the subway, and go to Princess Margaret Hospital. I drop my pants, put on a blue robe, and arrange myself in position on the table. The machine buzzes, shooting my knee with hard radiation. It then moves from below to above and does it again. Then I go back to work.

Emotionally, I rocket from calm to insane in an instant and back. I've realized a few things though. It sounds stupid, but I'm still surprised at how consistently traumatic this is. Maybe I thought I'd have a handle on it by now.

I've also realized that, despite how crazy this is, how out of control I get, this is not stronger than me. (Over the phone one night, Linda said, "It's just cells.") I've made sure I have a few people to remind me of that in a few months.

◆   ◆   ◆

One day, while walking toward the corner to catch the streetcar to go to work, I realized in a burst of joy, a joy that burned like the sun, that I did not feel any pain.

Early on, Peter had prescribed a fairly new, but kick-ass anti-inflammatory/painkiller called Celebrex. My drug plan covered most of the cost. The one thing about having cancer is that no one is shy about offering you painkillers. This new pill muted my pain, giving me some relief.

This particular day, there was no pain at all. For the first time in months, I wasn't limping. The realization struck like lightning. It didn't last though. By the time I reached work, the ache was back, but those moments of freedom were sheer bliss.

There were other changes. The swelling seemed visibly smaller. One day, I found I was able to go up the stairs into my apartment alternating right foot…left foot…right foot. That was something I hadn't been able to do in a long time.

The tumour seemed to be shrinking, something that could only be good. However, the spectre of the illness and the massive, overpowering thought I was going to lose a part of my body continued lurking in the shadows.

At this point, my visits to Dr. Wunder began occurring in only one place. I no longer visited the hall near his office, the fracture clinic, or any other place. I became a regular, frequent visitor to the sarcoma clinic.

◆   ◆   ◆

04*04*00

I saw Dr. Wunder today. Even he seemed surprised by the speed with which this is passing. I had yet another student today. After asking most of the same questions, he poked and prodded. Then Dr. Wunder came in. The student got a detailed description of the surgery and impending reconstruction.

And my stomach dropped. I guess somewhere, buried underneath everything, was the vain hope that he would find the radiation had changed things so much that it would render the surgery unnecessary. No such luck.

I know how lucky I am: how much worse this could be. But the thought of it suddenly fills me with dread.

◆   ◆   ◆

I had hoped. So lost in the daily routine, I allowed myself the luxury of fantasizing that the need for the surgery would somehow disappear. The radiation would miraculously kill all the tumour cells and regrow the destroyed tissue and bone. But hope can be a fickle thing. It can be crushed easily if the hope has been a vain one. There would be no eleventh-hour miracle. The damage was too great and irreversible. All would proceed as planned.

Then, in the midst of it all, my birthday came. It was the birthday that, so many years ago, I thought would leave me irretrievably old.

◆   ◆   ◆

Happy fucking birthday to me.

Woke up to an empty house, had a radiation treatment, saw Dr. Catton and I have an MRI in an hour and a half.

Yippee.

Dr. Catton noticed the swelling has gone down. He told me that, in about 20 percent of cases, they see this kind of dramatic response. When they do the surgery, they find the tumour is mostly dead.

I should find that comforting. I should feel that it shows the treatment is working. But I feel cheated.

I'm going to go through major surgery and reconstruction, followed by a long convalescence and physiotherapy over a tumour that may already be dead. In my head, I know it's a chance we can't take. They have to make damn sure it's gone.

The visions of what's going to be left of me when this is over dance in my head like a nightmare. The recurring thoughts of skin grafts and rearranged muscles chill me.

Now that the radiation is nearly over, there's nothing except the spectre of the scalpel to occupy my brain.

I'm scared, and there's no emotional refuge. Home is the place I have to take care of, keep clean, buy groceries for, and cook in because no one else will if I don't. Work is the place where I can barely keep on top of things and make mistakes.

That's all my life is—home and work. The boundaries of my world, like the edges of a flat earth, are someplace to fall off if I get too close.

Most times, it feels like I've gone over already.

◆   ◆   ◆

On a bright note, I came home one day shortly before my birthday and found a box waiting for me. My friends Beth and Mike had put together a care package for me. Mistakenly thinking I was in chemotherapy and therefore nauseated, Beth had baked a fabulous batch of ginger cookies because ginger is known to settle the stomach. There were holistic instructions for relieving nausea as well. There was also a bag of gummy spiders, and Mike had included a Beanie Baby cat. He also included a gift that touched me deeply, his copy of one of his favourite books, a science fiction paperback that had obviously been read dozens of times. The spine was cracked, and the covers were worn. His love for the book (and I guess, by extension, me) shone on every dog-eared page. The whole package brightened my day. For a short while, it actually held the darkness at bay.

On my actual birthday, Kerry took me for drinks and dinner to celebrate. We had a lovely time, just enjoying each other's company in a way we hadn't in a long time.

However, a new storm was brewing at work, one I was in no shape to deal with. Though I wasn't supposed to know, our head office had decided to close our store. While my radiation treatments were winding down and I was preparing for the six-week wait until my surgery, I was carrying the weight of the decision and my inability to share it with the staff I deeply cared about.

On April 12, five weeks after they began, my radiation treatments were over.

◆   ◆   ◆

04*12*00

It's late. I should be sleeping, but my head is buzzing.

It was my last radiation treatment today. I made it. The first part is over.

What a "full to the brim" day it was. I received a sweet card from Jenn, this cute teenage volunteer I've seen on and off over the five weeks. It was such a sweet gesture that I wanted to weep at her generosity. Then Scott from work, someone not given to displays of emotion of any kind, shook my hand and said congratulations.

It was Tracy's last day. Even though I'm not supposed to know, our head office is closing our store. Big secret! Don't tell!

In the evening, Carolyn took me to a charity reading of Alistair Macleod, Anne Marie Macdonald, and David Adams Richards. There were cocktails, hors d'oeuvres, readings, and book signings. Then, I stopped by to have a drink with Gordon at his work. (It's his birthday.)

Chock a block, slam-full day. My head is spinning. Could just be the cocktails.

Six
This I Believe...

◆

(With great admiration and respect to Robert Heinlein)

Many years ago, one of my favourite authors, Robert Heinlein, wrote an essay with the same title as the one above. He wrote of the beliefs that gave his life meaning, the values he held, and how they gave meaning and shape to his life. It's a wonderful piece of writing and a simple philosophy that, if adhered to by more people, could provide a foundation for a much better world. If you can find it, read it. It's in *Grumbles from the Grave* and in *Requiem* as well.

I don't think a person can go through something like this and not question the universe and his or her place in it and, by extension, the existence and nature of God. I know I did.

◆   ◆   ◆

03*07*00

In the constant whir of thoughts that this situation has begun, one great one persists. Until I found out about this, I wondered why I was here and what grand purpose my time in Toronto was for. I felt lost, having gone through the end of Kerry and me as lovers, uncertainty about work, etc.

Now, in this time of great crisis, I find I have been delivered into the hands of the best doctor in the country for this cancer and in the best hospital. I'm working for a company that, for the first time in my life, offers benefits that pay for my medications and a semiprivate room. Moreover, I work for someone who has gone through a similar thing at the same hospital.

I can't help but feel that I have been funnelled here. The universe has made sure I would be in exactly the right place when this happened. It's humbling that the gods have deemed me worthy of this protection and favour. I guess I now have to make good.

◆　　　◆　　　◆

For some, I think the experience of cancer must further entrench their atheism. "I am suffering, and the people around me are suffering. Therefore, God cannot exist because a God of love would never allow this to happen."

For others perhaps, their faith sustains them, giving them the hope and strength to face the hardships that a fight with cancer entails. They are in the hands of God at all times, and their faith sees them through. If the fight is eventually lost, then they are returning to the God who gave them life.

Perhaps others actually find their way to a faith that has been missing in their lives. Illness pushes them to find something in our world (and beyond it) that they have never seen before. I'm sure there are many subtle shades of faith along the way. There are as many different types of exploration as there are different people fighting the disease. And, believe me, one of the definite things I have learned is that there is no typical "person with cancer."

For me, as you can see in the previous journal entry, the questioning took the form of feeling that I had been delivered into the perfect blend of place and circumstances to deal with the trial of my cancer. It seemed my new life in Toronto had begun merely to place me in the hands of the professionals that could give me the best of care. Looking at this logically, there are huge holes in my reasoning. If just, kind fates are watching over me, why was I afflicted with the cancer in the first place? What was the initial incident in the chain? Was my entire relationship with Kerry just the mechanism to move me into position here?

These questions are the stuff that leads to madness. They are questions that rarely lead to answers, only theories. They are the stuff of faith, not logic. And faith is not logical.

I can tell you what I think about my relationship with God, Fate, or the Universe, but it is a purely subjective opinion. I don't pretend to have the keys to the kingdom. My answers and beliefs are my own, merely my own way of processing things that are unknowable, that is, the stuff of faith, not reason.

To begin, I do not believe we are merely the product of biological processes, that is, the random fusion of cells and the firing of neurons. I don't think Michelangelo, Beethoven, Gandhi, or Mother Theresa were mere genetic accidents. I

believe we all have the spark of magic in us and that spark lives on when the physical shell is gone.

What happens after our physical bodies die? I have no idea. I've never died so
I can't say what happens. Perhaps we join God in a paradise. Perhaps we return to
a primordial source of energy and consciousness that fuels the birth of new souls.
Perhaps we return to a new incarnation to perfect ourselves in a pursuit of Nir-
vana. I can't say. Deep down, I believe the magic of our individual souls is not
lost when we die. Somewhere and somehow, the great, conflicted, sometimes
weak beings we are continue.

The thing that has always bothered me most about most religions is the basic
assumption that there is some fundamental wrongness in us as human beings,
which the religion is duty bound to correct. I don't believe this. Every day, we are
bombarded with messages that tell us we are not good enough, attractive enough,
or spiritual enough. I think, even though people are often weak and capable of
stupidity and hurtfulness, we are also capable of great good and great acts of love
and kindness. Doing a bad thing is not the same as being a bad person. Our
actions in a given situation may be good or bad, but that does not take away from
our basic worth as human beings.

In terms of God, I don't think there is a bearded patriarchal father figure sitting in heaven, watching our actions and demanding we worship him. My feeling
is that God is more of a force, a power beyond our ability to grasp in many ways.
I think we see him/her/it when we sacrifice for another person. I believe I see it
when I see a sunset exploding in colours that takes my breath away. I see it in the
leaves in the fall. I believe I hear it in music that makes my spine tingle or moves
me to tears with its beauty. I see it in the faces of the people who love me, warts
and all. I know I see it in the people who brought me through my cancer and
saved my life.

Before I faced this disease, I don't know if I believed in Evil with a capital "E."
Now I think I do. I know it is an emotional, irrational response, but I see this disease and what it does as evil. It is indicative of a fundamental universal force that
destroys what we create.

Now, do I believe in a devil? Logically, I guess you would think, if I believe in
a god-type force, I would have to. If I believe this disease is evil, then it must have
been caused by something, right? In the same way I don't believe in a personified
God, I don't really believe in a horned Lucifer. I guess I believe mostly in the concept represented by the yin and yang symbol. Without light, there is no darkness.
Without destruction, there is no creation. What we perceive as evil is often the
result of greed and weakness, the baser emotions. These come from our weak-

nesses. They are our responsibility. Blaming our failings on an outside source is a dangerous trap.

I guess this leads to my next point—responsibility. How we respond to situations is our responsibility. My actions, choices, and decisions I make in response to my situation are my own. The consequences arising from them are mine as well. If I inadvertently cause pain to someone because of something I have done, that responsibility is mine. If my life is not what I wanted it to be, the responsibility is mine. My choices brought me to where I am.

Now, this may seem to fly in the face of my own earlier words about fate and its manipulation of me into the place I am. I acknowledge the paradox. The best answer I have to the inherent contradiction, I read in (of all things) a Superman novel written by Elliot S! Maggin. He wrote, "An electron that is part of an atom in an ocean may determine on which energy level it orbits, but it does not affect the coming and going of the tides." Somewhere between our free will and the tides of the universe is a line that divides the things we can control from the things we can't. I don't know where that line is. I have thought about it often and have concluded that I'll never know. I can only try like hell to change the things I can and accept the things I can't while accepting my successes and failures with as much grace as possible.

Perhaps, while we cannot always control what happens to us, we always have the responsibility for how we respond to it.

We are not perfect. God knows I'm not. I don't know if we even have the capacity for perfection within us, but I believe we have the capacity to be more than we are, that is, to be better than our baser instincts and negative emotions would have us behave.

What are my own principles? To start with, I use the golden rule: Do unto others as you would have them do unto you. Everything else springs from that. If you want people to be nice to you, be nice to them. It sounds like such a simple thing, so why is it so difficult to follow? If I knew the answer, I would be a wealthy, powerful man. Perhaps our society has become more and more competitive and less and less cooperative. There is a deep underlying feeling in our modern world that, if we grant something to another, be it a group or person, we have lost something ourselves. There are limited resources. Therefore, if someone else gets some, we have lost some. Maybe it's the socialist in me, but I think I would rather we all had some than I had a lot.

I believe in kindness. I believe that each day, in some small way, it is our responsibility to make the way a little easier for our fellow humans. Even if that something is as small as opening a door for someone or smiling and being friendly to a store clerk or a transit driver. I believe small kindnesses propagate and are passed on. In a world that is growing increasingly insane every day, I think they are sometimes our only weapon against the growing darkness. Each of us must keep the lights of hope and kindness alive. Will it change the course of nations? No. But it just might brighten someone's day and ease their passage through the hazards of day-to-day life. And that is a valid goal.

I believe in honesty. We must speak the truth about ourselves and our lives, especially those of us who live lives that differ from what is perceived to be the mainstream. Those who would believe we are a minority or are somehow wrong in our differentness must be made to see that we are here, our lives matter, and we will not go away in the name of conformity. I believe we must be honest with each other, even though we must always temper honesty with kindness and compassion. Too often, the truth is used as a weapon to bludgeon someone else as the speaker claims, "I was just being honest." We must speak the truth with love, not malice.

I believe we must learn to respect each other's differences. The fact that someone thinks differently than me doesn't make me right and him wrong. If we were all the same, the world would be an awfully dull place. Too often, people seem to think, because someone is different, be it a matter of religion, skin colour, or sexual orientation, they can then deny those people something. I don't care if someone thinks I'm going to burn in hell because I'm gay. I object to that person using their belief to deny me basic rights others enjoy. Having a belief is not wrong. Translating that belief into oppression is. I may not agree with what you say, but I'll vehemently defend your right to say it.

I believe there are many things worth dying for but few or none that are worth killing over. Would I have gone off to fight Hitler? I honestly don't know. I've never been in a situation where I've had to make that decision, and it's a moot point now. If I knew that giving my life would have a tangible benefit (that is, saving lives or preventing war), I'd like to think I would do it. Asking me to kill another person who, chances are, is not actually the person causing the problem but is just another pawn in the power struggle? I don't know. I suppose I would say there are times when killing might be necessary. (Maybe it's an absolute last resort.) It is never right, just, or correct.

I believe in forgiveness. Over the years, I have done many stupid, thoughtless, and cruel things as I acted from my weaknesses, fears, and rampant insecurities. In those situations, I hope the person I offended would forgive me. Therefore, I cannot legitimately refuse to forgive someone who has done the same to me. If I want to be forgiven, I must forgive.

Years ago, I heard a line on a TV show that has stayed with me. "The man who trusts can never be betrayed, only mistaken." I believe that is true. A person who betrays my trust is someone who will most likely find unhappiness littering his path. If I betray my principles by becoming bitter and resentful, I have lost something. It's the same with kindness, smiles, warmth, and compassion. If a person chooses to reject my offer of help, my smile, or my generosity, then they have lost, not me. Trust and kindness are worthy ideals to pursue whether they are ever returned or not. The exercise of warmth and generosity I aim for makes me feel good. I want to live in a world where people are decent and compassionate to each other. Maybe my actions can help bring us a bit closer to that world, even if only by a millimetre.

As I rant from my soapbox, I know how I must sound. I am a white, working-class male whose parents never beat him or used drugs or drank. I never went to school fearing for my life or worrying about gangs. I grew up in a country where I didn't have to worry about being shot, blown up, or tortured. Having cancer has been the worst thing I have ever experienced. I may sound hopelessly naïve to you. But the things I have written constitute the kind of person I want to be and the way I want to be treated. They are the goals I set for myself that I don't always reach. But I keep trying.

One of my friends from my McKim days, Paul Regehr, once said that trying your best to live a good life is the way to go because, no matter what, you win. If there is a reward waiting after death, you will be rewarded for the kindness and love you sowed in life. If there is nothing after death and we just cease, your life has been spent easing the path for those around you and inspiring them to do the same for you. Either one of those options sounds good, don't you think?

The truth is that we do not pass through this life without the assistance of other people. We can ease their path, or we can make it harder. They can do the same for us. I want to be one of those people who enrich the lives of others, who ease their journeys in some way, however small. I believe the world and I are better for it.

This I believe with all my heart.

Seven
Lull

A relative silence followed the end of the radiation. I underwent a six-week forced rest period. The radiation had damaged my tissues, hindering my body's ability to heal. I would need all of the recuperative powers I could muster after the surgery, so we had to allow time for my body to recover. While my body healed, life returned to a semblance of normalcy. I had time to ponder the other day-to-day crises of life.

The imminent closing of the store became known at a meeting, even though everyone had begun suspecting before the announcement was made. The company promised new positions would be found for us, so we all began considering where we might want to go.

For days, we went through the motions, doing our best to run the store and take care of our customers. Then our year-end rolled by, and the numbers on our P and L (Profit and Loss statement) were impressive. A phone call said we might not be closing after all. We waited in limbo until the reprieve eventually came through. The store would remain open, but we didn't find out until later. I spent a good chunk of my wait for surgery not knowing what was happening with the store. I didn't know what place there would be for me when all of the dust settled. I really had no idea what my abilities were going to be when I finally recovered. I tried factoring in possibilities, considering a change to our Internet group in some capacity, as I grew uncertain about my mobility and strength after the surgery. In the end, it just became something I couldn't worry about. The implications and stresses of just being a person with cancer took up all of my mental energy. Decisions of career became just another thing to deal with later.

◆   ◆   ◆

I rub aloe into the skin of my knee, trying to repair some of the skin damage the radiation caused. As my hands move over the joint, it's odd to contemplate that the joint won't be there six weeks from now.

   I keep having these "Oh shit" moments when the sheer normalcy of everything is replaced by that sudden, two-by-four to the forehead feeling of, "Oh my God, I have cancer, and I'm losing my knee to it in six weeks."

◆   ◆   ◆

The aloe became a ritual, as did long soaks in the bathtub with my left leg perched on the edge of the tub to keep the abused flesh of the knee out of the hot, bubbly water. I burned candles and listened to calming music. I went for walks constantly. The entire time, I wondered how long I wouldn't be able to and if I would ever walk normally again.

Eventually, Pauline returned from England. James finished his school year and returned home. One Saturday night, I went to a housewarming party being held by a couple I know. They had finally taken possession of a huge, gorgeous condo with a view of the lake. It proved to be an unusual evening in many ways. Other than Dave M. and Emily, I didn't know anyone there. I had heard of most of them because they were friends of my friend Kim. Though, in another of those postmodern twists, I was meeting them before Kim did. The Internet is such a strange and wonderful thing.

The party proved to be doubly surreal. Besides Dave M. and Emily, no one knew about my cancer. I didn't really know what to do. The cancer had accompanied me, as it did everywhere. Should I introduce it, or just leave it there, invisible at my side? I can be awkward in social situations at the best of times, and this only intensified the unease.

As the evening drew on, I found myself in conversation with another David, a friend of Dave and Emily's from Rochester, New York. Perhaps we gravitated to each other because we were the only single gay men there. I don't know, but we found ourselves thoroughly enjoying each other's company. Something just clicked, inspiring some good-natured whispering and finger-pointing. When it grew late, it just seemed to make sense to spend the night together. It was definitely what we both wanted. We retired to his hotel room.

Even though we did spend the night together, we mostly held each other. Now, I've never really been the "hold each other all night" type. There are always one too many arms in the way, and it's too hard to fall asleep. But it worked this time.

In those hours, I felt safe (as close to safe as I could feel in the circumstances) for the first time since the diagnosis and even earlier. There was no pressure or expectations. It was just comfortable and safe. In David, I found a respite, a haven of the comfort I often longed for in my journal. He came to visit once more, driving up on Monday night. For brief seconds, I entertained thoughts of a bourgeoning relationship. The truth was, beyond the fact that he lived in New York, he soon got a job in Minneapolis. We were both too smart to think there was anywhere it could go.

Over the Easter weekend, the first of the summer support visits began. When Kerry met Ken, I told him I couldn't handle having Ken around the house with everything happening. Kerry had been involved in a couple of short, tempestuous relationships in the period since the previous fall, causing a huge amount of tension and drama in the house. Though Ken would eventually prove to be a serious, long-term relationship, I wasn't able to go through more of the trauma that had characterized much of our autumn and winter. I don't know if I had any right to ask, and I don't know if it was right or wrong. But, at the time, I felt I did not have a choice. Kerry began spending all of his time with Ken. He was all but living there in every sense without an official address change. His bed was empty here, and that gave us a place for guests.

Margot Keeler, one of my dearest friends from my high school creative writing class, was the first to make plans to come. As soon as that was arranged, my sister, Sue, said she could come at the same time. Our house was full, but we enjoyed ourselves. Margot slept in Kerry's bed. My sister volunteered to take the couch. (It was an amazingly comfortable couch.)

Sue arrived around noon on Saturday, April 22. Margot's plane came in around 4:00 PM. She had travelled to see me on her birthday. That evening, we went to a little Indian restaurant on Queen Street. Margot and Pauline were far more knowledgeable about Indian cuisine, so Sue and I just sort of sat back and let them order. We feasted on onion bhaji, lamb biryani, paneer and peas, and many other delicacies before staggering home, completely satisfied.

On Easter Sunday, we cooked a wonderful, completely untraditional Easter dinner of poached ginger salmon, couscous, and green beans with orange and almonds. Then we drank wine and curled up with a stack of decorating magazines, showing each other pictures we liked. Kerry's boyfriend, Ken, got us free passes to the Egyptian exhibit at the Royal Ontario Museum, so we spent an afternoon prowling in and out of the various rooms. I showed them my neighbourhood. We watched the news channel with the sound down, laughing hysterically at the crazy mistakes in the closed captioning. (Jesus Christ became Juice Cease Christ. Janet Reno became January Reno.)

At one point, we were watching a music channel. A Reba McEntire video came on. A stark image of a young mother appeared, pulling off a wig to reveal a head of hair that was patchy and uneven from chemotherapy. My sister, sixteen years my senior, just slid over to me and slipped her arm around me. I could see the beginnings of tears in her eyes.

Early Tuesday morning, she left for home. Margot and I had a few more days before she had to leave as well. We were in a vintage furniture store, and I saw a beautiful, stripped metal bed frame from the 1940s. I fell in love with it, and we walked around a bit more while I felt angst about it. Finally, I knew I really wanted it. On some level, I figured, for the amount of time I was going to spend in bed, I should have a nice one. Also, it was important to have something nice, a major purchase that was mine after the dividing of the property from my relationship with Kerry. When the time came for me to pay for it, Margot gave me half. She just handed it to me because she knew it was something I needed. We carried it home while I limped and she carried the majority of the weight. We then put it together. On Thursday, she was gone as well.

◆   ◆   ◆

04*30*00

I have a small scar on my left knee. I've had it since I was a child. It's about an inch or two long. I vaguely remember scraping it and picking the scab off. It's been there forever. I caught a glimpse of it today while rubbing aloe into the stressed skin. I realized, once this is over, it probably won't be there anymore. Perhaps the larger scars that will be present will swallow it. It was such a small thing in the face of everything else, and I still feel a pang at the thought of its absence.

◆   ◆   ◆

The days of waiting passed, both agonizingly slowly and far too fast at the same time. Somewhere in this time, I discovered Martina McBride's CD, *Emotion*. As I so often do with new music, I find something new and fall in love like a new lover. I listen to it (and only it) repeatedly, plumbing the depths of what it says to me until I'm sick of it. One song, "From the Ashes," became the theme song for what I was feeling then. It's a song about rebirth and the decisions we are sometimes forced to make to leave what we know and make a drastic change. The imagery of being reborn from the ashes filtered deep into my consciousness, even though the changes I was soon to go through were not of my making.

◆   ◆   ◆

05*04*00

The walls of my world are burning down. I have no doubt that I will emerge, phoenixlike once it's all over, but I just don't know who I'll be and what the world will look like.

My physical body is going to be permanently changed. My emotional self is being permanently changed. People I thought were friends have fallen away after disappointing me gravely. My store may be gone by the time I heal. Even if it isn't, my days in there are over. I may have a job at the Internet group or I may be unemployed.

I just don't know what's going to be left. On some days, I'm sick to death of putting on a brave face. I just want to be comforted just once. I want to pillow on a comforting shoulder.

◆   ◆   ◆

At my regular appointment at the sarcoma clinic, I received my surgery date, May 24. I discussed more details with Dr. Wunder and one of the residents on his team. (Gordon was there and had more presence of mind to ask more questions than I did.) I then went to the preadmission unit.

I filled out all of the necessary paperwork, including next of kin, insurance number for semiprivate room, and such. Blood was taken, and I was given pamphlets on the pain control methods to be used.

Like a woman in labour, I was to have an epidural to block the pain and patient-controlled analgesia (PCA) pump that would allow me some control over the painkillers. Elizabeth, the nurse who took my blood and vital signs, asked the question I would come to hear many times during my stay in the hospital. "On a scale of zero to ten, zero being no pain at all and ten being the worst pain you've ever felt, how would you rate your pain?"

I confessed I wasn't sure I'd know how to answer because I had little to compare it to. With slightly widened eyes, she looked at me and said, "Trust me, when you hit ten, you'll know. And you probably will."

Okay.

When the appointment was over, I collected Gordon from the waiting area. He was feverishly working on rewrites of his most recent play that would be given a public reading in a few weeks. Thanks to this meeting with Elizabeth, I would spend much less time in admitting on the morning of the surgery, which was good because the surgery was scheduled for 8:00 AM.

◆   ◆   ◆

05*11*00

Well, I have my surgery date. May 24.

Oh, fuck.

I've been feeling like that a lot lately. I've been going along, and, all of a sudden, I feel like all of the breath in my body has been sucked out of me.

As Gordon said the other day, "This is Act 2."

◆   ◆   ◆

When I sat down to write this next passage, to relate the story of those final days leading up to my surgery, I procrastinated even more than I usually do. I spent an hour or so reading instead of sitting down to work. The nearer I got to the actual event, the nearer I came to the physical and emotional trauma of the operation that would forever alter my life and my relationship with the world. I could feel my own resistance to reliving the long recuperation and the indignities and helplessness of the days that would follow. Like the implacable quality of the cancer itself, the realities of what happened cannot be avoided. The memories of those days, that time of pain and slow recovery, cannot be dismissed. So I gritted my teeth and called forth the memories.

Several months before the surgery, I met a man named Michael at the store. I saw him browsing more than once, and he caught my attention. I found him attractive and, in my newfound singleness, attempted to engage him in conversation. On those first occasions, contact was quite superficial. He didn't seem all that interested initially. My rampant sexiness or anything had not bowled me over.

One evening, he came in looking for a specific set of books for his nephew. I was able to track some down and order them. After he left, I realized one of the books wasn't available until a few months later, so I called the number he left to leave a message. The outgoing message contained another man's name as well. It was obvious they were more than roommates. I thought, "Too bad for me." I then let it go.

Several weeks later, the books came in. He picked them up on one of my days off. One of my coworkers said he had come in and expressed his gratitude.

I next saw him two weeks before my surgery. We chatted briefly, and he thanked me again for ordering the books. I had to go to the back room, and it occurred to me that I should let him know I was going to be gone for a while. I had been slowly informing my regular customers, and he was a nice person. I felt a kinship to him, as I felt to the other people who helped form the boundaries of my work world. By the time I came back onto the sales floor, he was gone.

I thought I might not see him again until I came back to work, if ever. But fate had another twist up its sleeve.

◆   ◆   ◆

<u>05*15*00</u>

On Friday night, I decided to go out for a drink after work. At Woody's, I ran into a man I've talked to at the store, Michael. I spent the evening talking with him and his friend Brian. I told him about my cancer and the impending surgery. When we left, a thunderstorm was going on, so Michael offered to drive me home. We talked about my situation with Kerry, and he told me he was in the dying days of a relationship. Due to his father's serious illness, he wasn't able to deal with it.

When we reached my place, he admitted he was attracted to me. I told him I felt the same way. He said, during his nap before coming out, he had dreamed about meeting me at the bar. We both knew we weren't in a position to do anything about it. We both had way too much on our plates, but there was a strong current of desire. So we kissed—deep, passionate kissing. He said he felt a bit guilty.

I came in, and he went home. He said he'd try to call me the next day. Typical of my timing, he called during the exact half hour I was out for a walk. That night, I had three e-mails from him.

I was swept away on a wave of longing for this to be the beginning of something. Even if it had to wait for things to be sorted out with my knee and his father, at least the emotional something would be there.

But he came by the store today, after having been wracked with guilt about this. And we had "the talk." We can only be friends, etc.

I know he's right. There's too much going on now., and deep inside, I know my feelings, though real, are coming from all the wrong places.

I just can't handle being alone in the dark with the demons. While I know everyone else has feelings and pain about this, I'm the only one going through this alone. Kerry goes home to Ken. Gordon goes home to David. But here in the brooding dark, there's only me.

I just wanted a shoulder to lean on that was mine.

◆   ◆   ◆

As you can see, these thoughts, this abiding feeling of loneliness, followed me constantly. It crept through my heart and, as such, into journal entries repeatedly. It was worst in the dark, once the day was over and I was tucked in bed alone. There is no shield against those thoughts then.

I've thought a lot about the benefits of being single or being in a relationship during a time like this. Obviously, someone who loves you and shares his or her life with you would be a great source of strength in the dark times. He or she would be someone to shoulder the weight in the moments when you can't do it yourself. Friends can do that, but, for the most part, they live somewhere else. In the dark, late at night or after the friends have returned home, the demons come calling. A partner is the one who will be with you in those odd hours.

Months later, when I met Mike Forbes, his boyfriend Skip slept on the floor beside Mike's bed the night before his surgery. Many times, I would have given my soul for someone who would have done that for me without being asked, someone who would just have known that I needed it.

The thought of what this might do to a relationship persists. There are few more stressful experiences than a life-threatening illness, and that stress is going to have an effect on a relationship. For all this fight did to me, it was mine alone. My fortunes rose and fell in direct proportion to it. I can imagine the helplessness felt by those who loved me, unable to do much more than watch and support.

In the end, I suppose it's moot. I was single when this happened and stood through the storm without a partner beside me. Instead, I had true, loyal friends. And I'm still standing.

◆   ◆   ◆

Some days, I look into the abyss that is this disease, the black hole of cancer and its corona of laden emotion. I see…nothing.

My strength fails me. When I try taking stock of the resources I will need to get through the hell that is to come, there's nothing. Just nothing. And I wonder just how I will get through this.

I laid awake the other night until 2:00 AM, brooding about the details: things such as how will I get my underwear over the bandages. I wear boxer briefs, you see, tight in the legs. Will it be difficult to get them on? What about showering? I spent a good five minutes on Saturday contemplating the logistics of getting into a claw-foot bath-tub with only one weight-bearing leg. The myriad problems swell before me like a wall of black water. How am I ever to surmount them?

The prospect of being practically an invalid for a substantial period disturbs me. I have always had a prideful, stubborn streak. I have always been torn between needing and needing to never need anything from anyone. I yearn for comfort. Yet, on some level, the desire repulses me. I must keep the armour in place.

I'm so tired. I can see dark circles forming under my eyes, and I know the long fight back hasn't even started.

◆   ◆   ◆

This feeling of not wanting to appear I needed anything wasn't new. I've always been that way. I think it comes from learning to be gay when and where I did. For too long, I lived with the stigma something was inherently wrong with me. My response to it was constantly striving to be better, stronger, and nicer than everyone else so people would like me and forgive my flaw. Even though those feelings of inherent inferiority have passed, the patterns of dealing with things have not. I still keep much of my pain inside, trying to be the "best little boy in the world." (This is a tip of the hat to Andrew Tobias, writing as John Reid.) That went on until I was diagnosed with cancer. The tide of emotions brought about by the illness battled their way through my restraints. There was no choice except releasing them. Friends saw me weep with rage and frustration. They saw my deep fear as well. These were friends I never showed this side of myself to.

I have learned to verbalise more. I talk endlessly about my feelings in relation to this struggle, prying open the experience to understand. I remember the social worker stopping by after the surgery and saying something about how men tend to hold their emotions in and not speak. I told him this wouldn't be a problem for me. But, as usual, it was somewhat of a lie.

◆ ◆ ◆

05*17*00

Well, there you go. I've taken to telling a waitress about my cancer, just to have some-one to tell about it and talk to about it. I'm an ailment whore.

The waitress in question was a cutie though. She looked all of twelve. She was dressed in black with a pierced tongue. Yet, she had this cherubic, angel face that com-pletely contradicted everything else. Her reaction was sweet though. She did not give me any pity or drama. She just provided a wide-eyed, "I didn't know that." It was kind of refreshing.

Illness-land is a fucking boring place to be sometimes. This all-consuming monkey on the back colours everything. The constant pain, fear, and feelings of being on the end of a plank alone with the wolves gathering. Perhaps that should be sharks. Mustn't mix metaphors.

But why not? What are the rules anymore? To borrow from Rent, *"When your own blood cells betray." What are the foundations?*

Friendship: *those relationships that hold on despite all challenges. Not the fly-by-nights or also-rans that fall away. The Gordon-Margot-Kerry-Carolyn-Landon friends.*

Strength: *often in short supply. What there is is often stretched to its breaking point.*

Grace: *often a tough one as well when fatigue and pain set in. Even harder when dread rises up before you, blocking your path.*

Dignity: *another tough one when you're arranged on a radiation rig in a skimpy robe, shitting into a bedpan, or babbling from pain meds. No, dignity's the first one to go.*

◆ ◆ ◆

05*20*00

I suddenly find myself feeling totally gypped, which is odd because I've always really known that life is unfair.

I came here with Kerry, thinking I would spend the rest of my life with him. That fell apart, and I felt stranded here. I was just getting to feel good about myself again, have sex again, and feel as if someone might feel something for me again. And this happens. Talk about a raw deal.

Now there's a whole new set of shit to deal with, not the least of which is feeling attractive again (with massive scars down my leg). I deserve something good now, but I suppose I have to come back to the fact that this could be so much worse. There's just no telling how this is going to play out though.

I hate this endless waiting, yet I still just want Wednesday to never come.

◆   ◆   ◆

Family was missing from the list of foundations mentioned in that journal entry. I talked with them often. My sister Sue had visited to lend support. One night, my sister Linda said, regardless of the cost, she would be here with me when I went into surgery. My parents weren't able to be here because they had already made arrangements to travel to Alaska with a relative from England. (They came to see me once I was out of the hospital.) True to her word, Linda arrived on the afternoon of Sunday, May 21.

We had a few days to spend together to just wander. We went shopping for clothes for her, and I convinced her to buy a slinky, stretchy white dress she didn't think she could get away with. Like I had done with Sue, I took her to the Royal Ontario Museum. We couldn't get in to see the special Egyptian exhibit, which was sold out on its last day, but we looked at the animals, gemstones, and minerals. (She made a beeline for the gems!) We looked at the Chinese exhibit. We ate dinner at my favourite Chinese place on the corner, which was cheap and excellent. I go there when I don't feel like cooking. The entire time, we did not talk about it. We did not let the cancer intrude on the first time we had spent together in more than a year.

◆   ◆   ◆

05*23*00

Tomorrow. Bright and early. 8:00 AM. Surgery. Admissions at 6:30 AM. Six-and-a-half hours later, cancer gone. The old knee gone, new knee in.

Linda's here, being brave. So am I. I caught a glimpse of moisture in her eyes. As I write this, I feel it in mine.

There's no escape now. It's here—an end to the cancer and a beginning to the long healing. What I wouldn't give to have those strong, broad shoulders to hold me right about now.

Everyone else seems to be more messed up about this than me. Kerry was a wreck the other night. Pauline says she's a wreck, but her surface seems calm. Gordon is being tough and loving. Nothing shows through the cracks. At work, Margot hugged me. She never hugs.

◆　　　◆　　　◆

The morning of the surgery, all of us were up at an ungodly hour. I think I woke around 4:00 or 5:00 AM. Fear knotted my stomach. The car wreck was upon me. The car's frame was buckling from the pressure, and the windows were shattering. The wait was coming to an end. I would know soon enough how bad the crash would be, how severe the casualties would be. All of us were quiet as we took our turns in the shower and calmly got in the taxi that took us to the hospital. Only occasional nervous laughter broke the silence. I reported to admissions. After checking in, I waited with the others. Each of us had a small bag of essentials brought from home. We watched the clock and waited as others were served. Kerry joined us, neatly wearing his suit for work. When it was my turn, I was directed to the eleventh floor. There, the floor nurse took me to a room. As it turned out, it was not mine. There was some delay in preparing it. I changed into another skimpy hospital gown and waited to be taken down. When the time came, my entourage followed me to the surgical floor. I surrendered my glasses. Dr. Wunder was there, and everyone met him. I then met the anaesthetist and the scrub nurse. Their names are lost, sucked into the paralysis of my fear. I said good-bye to everyone and was wheeled into the operating room.

I have no real impressions of the operating room other than it being cold and bright. People were bustling around. Someone asked me to sit up so he could insert the epidural. As I sat up, my gown opened and basically fell off.

The last thing I remember is sitting on the edge of the table, practically buck naked, with hands at the small of my back.

Eight
Surgery

The next seven hours of my life are gone, a void in which my whole relationship to the world and my own body would change. The next thing I remember is waking up in the recovery room, stoned to the gills and unable to see anything except blurs.

I've done a bit of research since then, asking questions of people who were either there or had seen a similar procedure. I've even watched a bit of orthopaedic surgery on television, even though my tolerance for filmed operations has decreased a lot since experiencing it myself. I do know this. What Peter once told me is true. Orthopaedic surgery is carpentry. It is incredibly sophisticated carpentry. Bone and muscle are substituted for wood, but it is definitely carpentry, involving hammers, saws, screws, and the like. Jon Hunter, the psychiatrist I would eventually see, told me, when he did his surgical rotation on orthopaedics, he was performing a procedure and looked down to see that the drill in his hand was Black & Decker. I'm glad my knowledge of what follows is secondhand.

At some point after the epidural was in place, I would have gone under. I don't know exactly when. I hope I was laid out first in order to spare the team the task of manhandling me into place. Once I was unconscious, I was arranged into position. The anaesthetist would likely have taped my eyes shut to protect them from any accidental damage.

I would then have been intubated. The anaesthetics are neuralepts, which would depress my ability to breathe on my own. Intubation allows them to monitor and control my breathing. At this point, I was also catheterized.

Two or three times, while the residents were shaving and washing my leg, Dr. Wunder checked the MRI and CT. He measured the tumour and determined where to make his incisions and how much to remove. Markings were possibly made on the leg as guidelines.

Once the leg was clean, a stretchy, sticky plastic was wrapped around it to prevent the skin from tearing while the leg was open. The skin was stretched to allow them to work.

The initial incision was made, encompassing the biopsy site. Because the biopsy needle infiltrated the tumour, there was a possibility that tumour cells may have moved along the needle's path. Removal of that path minimizes the risk.

The removal of the tumour would have then begun, taking all of the affected tissue in one piece. It sounds simple, doesn't it? In my case, consider the tumour had affected the knee joint, including the back of my kneecap, my quadriceps muscle, and the lower portion of my femur. All of the affected areas would have to be removed in one lump, including a two-centimetre margin of healthy tissue around it. The various cut ends of things moved aside would then have to be kept track of. I can't even keep track of my keys for more than ten minutes. I can't even imagine having the concentration and focus to perform a task like this.

The last thing removed would have been bone, including the removal of the back of the patella. In my case, the amount of bone that had to be removed corresponded almost exactly to the bone that was radiated. This made things easier because the radiated bone with its inhibited healing would not have taken the prosthesis well. Once the tumour was completely removed, it was sent to the lab to determine if the margins were clean. Mine were. If they hadn't been, more tissue would have been taken.

Once the margins were declared clean, preparations were made for the implantation of the prosthesis. The marrow canals of the femur and tibia were made larger to accept the anchors of the prosthesis, which were the first pieces to be implanted.

A Kotz prosthesis is designed to be modular. (I've seen pictures!) Pieces are custom fit together to be exactly the right size for each patient. The image that promptly came to mind was that of a large Tinkertoy. (I know it is somewhat blasphemous.) The final pieces put in place would have been the connecting segments of the hinge and the polyethylene bushing that attached them, somewhat like an axle.

To promote healing and replace the chunk of muscle removed in the surgery, a further incision was made in the outer part of my calf. A flap of calf muscle, the gastrocnemius, was cut at the lower end and flipped up. It was then sutured in place to cover the outside edge of the prosthesis. This provided a barrier between the metal and the skin that would be grafted to replace what had been lost and provide healthy, nonradiated tissue to aid the healing of the graft. All the various ends were then sutured up, and two drain tubes were put in place.

The next step would have been the skin graft. I have seen this performed on TLC. First, the skin is harvested from the donor site with a device resembling an electric cheese slicer. A thin layer is removed and put through a machine, like a hand-operated pasta maker, that punches waffle-like holes in it. This allows the graft to cover an area up to two times as large as the donor site. More can be covered with less. As the graft heals, the holes grow in. Over the donor site, a stiff dressing aptly called a scarlet red was applied. As the graft donor site healed, the rigid edges would dry and slowly peel away.

Finally, there are staples—lots and lots of staples. Linda did a rough count and figured there were about a hundred in there, running down the eighteen-inch length of the incisions and around the edge of the skin graft. The leg was then dressed with a Jones bandage with rigid plaster along the bottom and mounds of padding along the top. After that, I was extubated and moved to recovery.

Nine
Hospital

While I was in surgery, Linda waited. Despite my assurances that she should go out and do something because the surgery would take hours, she waited. Pauline stayed for a while, left for work, and returned later in the afternoon. Gordon came at some point and waited with Pauline while Kerry took Linda for lunch. He then had to go see his father, who was at the airport passing through town. I was eventually taken to recovery, and they were informed. Linda called my parents to let them know I was all right.

The first thing I remember is the dim blur that was my first glimpse of the recovery room. They keep the lights low. Without my glasses, there was little to see except shadows. Once they realized I was awake, they checked on me and asked about my pain. At that moment, I was so doped up that I did not feel any pain at all. Everything felt disconnected, unreal, and dreamlike. When they asked if I could move my good leg, I couldn't. Of course, that didn't bother me. In my drug-addled state, nothing bothered me. Apparently, it concerned them. I was kept in recovery for a couple of extra hours to make sure nothing was seriously wrong. My epidural was dialled down. The control and sensation in my other leg returned. I think Dr. Wunder came and talked to me at some point, but my memories of that time are quite hazy.

I was returned to my room, travelling in a fancy, air-cushioned bed. I remember the occasional hiss as it altered the pressure against my body, which was designed to prevent bed sores from being in bed for an extended period. I spent five days in that bed with my leg wrapped in the massive Jones bandage. Two Hemovac drain tubes came from my leg. I also had a catheter, an IV of antibiotics, and an epidural. With five tubes and connections going in and out of my body, I felt like a Borg. I wasn't even one of the nasty, threatening Borg. I was more like one of the broken ones that has his vital bits salvaged and is then left behind. The scarlet red dressing was stiff against the graft donor site. The raw, scraped flesh underneath it pulsed with an acid sting.

When I roused back to consciousness, I met the nurse who would care for me for the first few days. Glenda was a sweetie with a Newfie accent you'd need a knife to cut through. Linda and Pauline were allowed to come and see me. Apparently, I was lucid enough to respond when spoken to, but was I pretty dopey. Pauline says I was "so cute." I answered questions posed to me, but only briefly. I couldn't form questions or complex answers. I would just lapse into silence. Eventually, they left me to sleep. They stopped at the Riverside Bistro on Queen Street for food and wine.

I slept fitfully that night, mostly because the nurses were in and out several times to check my vital signs and give me medications. The physical pain was a dull throb. When I was conscious, the emotional pain consisted of a deep, heartsick loneliness in the dark with only a few transplanted objects from home to keep me company.

The morning after the surgery, I experienced a succession of horrible pains in the muscle flap under the skin graft. In rapid sequence, spasms ran through the rearranged muscle, hitting at least an eight or nine on the pain scale. Thankfully, they passed after about five minutes. When I told Glenda, she passed the message along to the pain control team, who then increased the epidural to spare me from enduring it again.

I was able to eat the next morning. I had been warned that might be problematic. Many people experience nausea when they're taking morphine derivatives. Thankfully, I wasn't one of them. My appetite was fairly normal by the second day. They even started bringing the menu around so I could choose my meals for the next day.

I don't remember a lot from those first few days. There are a lot of gaps in my memory. I remember the pills. Every four hours, a nurse had my meds. Because of the constipating effects of the pain drugs, I took a stool softener. To help prevent blood clots, I took a blood thinner. There were extra pain pills. If I couldn't sleep at night, I took Ativan. Ten o'clock...two o'clock...six o'clock...ten o'clock...two o'clock. My vital signs, temperature, blood pressure, and pulse were taken several times a day. I remember this as the beginnings of the precise routines that would shape my days for the following weeks and months.

I watched TV when I could focus. I don't remember most of what I watched. I mostly saw the Food Network, HGTV, and reruns of *Bewitched*. In a corner of my mind, I knew I was just waiting, biding my time until I would see "it." Everyone came to visit again. Between visits, if not during, I napped.

Every time my visitor left, I wanted to scream for them to stay and sleep on the floor or in the chair beside my bed. I wanted anything to not be left alone in the dark again.

Kerry came that Thursday and said he had something for me. Reaching in his briefcase, he pulled out a Backstreet Boys CD. I said, "Haven't I suffered enough?" He looked at me and said, "You're missing the point." Then he pulled out a new Discman. He'd bought it because he knew how much I loved music and what a powerful force it was for me. Whatever other faults the man has, he is a real sweetheart when he wants to be.

The day after, I was moved to another room for some arcane hospital reason I still don't understand. I didn't object because the new room was great. It was larger and located on a corner of the building with huge windows on two walls. I arrived, and no one else was there because the other occupant, a teenage boy, had been given a weekend pass. I had the room to myself for nearly three days. At night, I could watch the glittering lights of downtown Toronto. I found them, the lit rooms and neon hotel signs, comforting. I don't really know why. Perhaps they were just a sign that there was life beyond my hospital bed and outside my four walls. Looking at those lights kept the dark at bay and made me feel less alone. They were signs there was something to the world that wasn't that room or that bed.

There's a picture of me that Kerry took during that first weekend. I mentioned something about wanting pictures of this experience. He brought in his camera and took some. There's one that chilled me when I saw it. I look gaunt and pale. There isn't even a trace of happiness or joy in my face. It's like someone turned me off; like my spirit had left my body. I don't recall feeling that way, but the picture haunts me to this day.

There were some lovely moments in those first few days, despite the initial oppressive weight of recovery. Kelly sent a beautiful bouquet of flowers. I received a visit from my boss, Margot, and her husband, Dennis. Even Goretti, the girl who managed the Second Cup where I had gone for my coffee every day, came to see me. The Monday after the surgery, Michael visited as well. I vamped and played the plucky survivor to mask my pain and the growing terror of what I would eventually see.

I realized how out of whack my body chemistry was when I tried putting my jewellery back on that weekend. I thought my rings and neck chain would make me feel a little more like myself. Within a day, they were turning black against my skin.

I could start bathing that weekend. Each day, the nurse brought a tub of water, a clean cloth, and a new gown. She then pulled the curtain. I sloshed awkwardly around the tubes all over my body. It would be literally months before I showered again.

To add insult to injury, at one point in those early, bed-ridden days, I had to have a suppository and use a bedpan. Believe me, those are words I never want to hear again as long as I live. For someone like me, for whom bodily functions are a matter of extreme privacy and something that is never discussed, being perched on a plastic pan and then having my butt wiped by someone I barely knew was uncomfortable and embarrassing beyond words. I burned with shame at it. Being unable to even clean myself was the ultimate helplessness. My already tortured dignity was stressed to breaking. I avoided using the pan again for as long as I could, but nature eventually won out. This time, the lucky nurse was a black woman I never saw again. She was quite serious until I expressed my feelings about the whole experience. She then smiled and told about being in a hospital in her teens and needing to use a bedpan. The nurse who brought it was a rather attractive man, and she felt completely humiliated. She just patted my shoulder and said, "I know how you feel."

Over the course of those five days, I was gradually disconnected from various tubes and drains. Doses of Percocet every four hours replaced the pain control pump and the epidural. (More pills!) The Hemovac tubes were taken out, and the catheter was removed. I was somewhat dreading the last, but the nurse did it at six o'clock in the morning. She came in with my pills, woke me, deflated the little balloon holding it in place, and slid it out. I thought, "Ow! Ow! Ow!" I then rolled over and went back to sleep. It couldn't have been *that* painful. Finally, the only remaining thing was the IV. The direct connection was replaced with something called a saline lock, a valve that goes into the vein like an IV but allows the IV line to be detached when not in use. The only downside is that the saline locks are only stable for a few days and then have to be moved. By the end of the second week, I had small, healing holes on my hands, wrists, and forearms.

At the beginning of the second week of my hospital stay, Dr. Wunder and his crew of residents (whom, because I was rarely introduced to them, I always thought of as the Wunderettes) came to open the bandage and see how I was healing. Two of them attacked the Jones bandage with scissors. I felt a surge of panic at the sight of them sawing away and peeling back the thick wads of padding. Once the remnants of the bandage were cleared away, Dr. Wunder took a close look and said, "It looks good."

I thought he was insane.

In that second, I realized the huge schism between what he meant and what I would have meant with the same phrase.

My leg was purple with bruising and swollen all the way down. The incision began at the midpoint of my outer thigh and travelled downwards. A ropy knot of newly forming scar was at the top edge of the skin graft, just above what looked like a cavernous divot where the edges of the graft divided. The graft itself was about four inches wide and nearly six inches long. It was pink with pebbled flesh. I could only think of the pictures I had seen of experiments performed on monkey brains. I don't know if you've ever seen them, but the scientists opened the monkeys' skulls and attached electrodes to stimulate various areas of the brain. The skin graft looked like one of those exposed monkey brains. The muscle flap looked bulbous under the grafted skin. The swelling made it look even worse. Around the edge of the graft was a turned-under ridge where the graft itself was attached to the radiation-ravaged skin of my knee, a pucker of scar that just emphasized the protrusion of the muscle flap. The lower edge of the skin graft came together into a Y. The incision line extended down my calf and ended about five inches from my ankle. The entire wound was held together by that line of nearly a hundred staples. It looked to me as if a shark had attacked me.

I fell apart after Dr. Wunder and his entourage were gone. In a haze of horror, I phoned Gordon. Later, he said he took the call in his home office in his underwear. He listened as I wept. My heart was torn raw.

When something like that faces you, you can intellectualize it. You think you've accepted the inevitability of your destiny. But, when it hits you in the face, like a fist that jars the very bones of your skull, your calm acceptance disappears. My life and my body were ruined.

That day, I wrote in my journal that the incision was three feet long, which was an exaggeration. When I was finally able to measure it, it was only eighteen inches. In those initial few days, it was monumental to me.

It was horrifying to see. Everyone told me it didn't look that bad. To me, it was hideous. All my fears of being maimed or ugly in some profound new way came rushing back to me. How could anyone ever love me again? What man would ever find me desirable with this thing where my leg had once been? I didn't have answers. When Gordon, Pauline, or Linda tried reassuring me, I nodded and pretended to believe their assurances while feeling mutilated and grotesque deep inside.

I kept up my usual façade, or I at least made a brave stab at it. I tried saving my tears and deep grief for the moments I was alone. I tried putting on the brave, stiff upper lip face whenever I had visitors.

To be honest, despite my dark feelings, there were plenty of times when we had a lot of fun. We laughed a lot, although I couldn't tell you at what. We took any opportunity for a little humour. Gordon brought CDs, including Tina Turner and the Pet Shop Boys. Kerry brought Ace of Base. My friend Roger brought a wallet full of Mike Oldfield. For my entertainment, I was brought munchies and cheesy magazines. Kerry brought a Wonder Woman magnet that went on the metal locker by my bed. A few days later, Gordon brought a Batgirl one to match.

With the Jones bandage gone, I was introduced to what would take its place, the Zimmer splint, a padded cloth, Velcro, and metal creation that would be used to keep my leg straight and somewhat protected in the months to come. Grey and rigid with a spongy pad behind the knee, the Zimmer was slid under my gently lifted leg and strapped closed. My leg was manipulated like a log or a slab of meat, something not alive anymore. I wasn't allowed out of bed without the splint, and it stayed on my leg constantly for three months. It was only removed for dressing changes.

Around this time, I got a new roommate. The young boy on the weekend pass returned just long enough to pack up his things and leave. His mother apologised for not stopping to become acquainted. Apparently, he'd had a rough day. I felt badly and tried reassuring her that I took no offence. Shortly after their departure, my new roommate was wheeled in after undergoing surgery. Dave Gripe was a twenty-year survivor of osteosarcoma. In the last year or so, the repair job on his hip had broken down. He had come from Rochester, New York, with his wife, Riki, to have what was called a revision. His hip and thigh were rebuilt with bone from the bone bank, which was bound together with wire and would eventually ossify like my prosthesis. When he roused from his postoperative grogginess, we hit it off. Riki was a singer, so I made sure to introduce her to David, Gordon's partner and my former roommate. They talked about singing for a long time while Dave and I just sat back and smiled. Whenever we could, we pulled back the curtains between our beds, which the nurses were always drawing, and created what I called the party room. Riki had to drive back and forth to Rochester to look after their children and to work, so I happily shared my circle of loving cheerleaders with Dave when she was gone.

I had a string of nurses in those days, too many to recall all of their names. Pat was a sweet maternal type with a trace of an accent that I think was Jamaican. Jane was barely out of nursing school when I met her. I remember sitting in the dark talking to her with my comforting tableau of lights beyond the windows. There was the pair I met only once, whose names are now lost to me. They had taped pictures of Mariah Carey and Whitney Houston over their own pictures on their hospital IDs. Sami was one of the two male nurses I had. I think he was Filipino, and he had a sweet, soft-spoken manner. Every time Pauline was there and he was changing the dressing on my leg, he was always concerned that she was okay.

For the most part, I found it interesting that, with the exception of Sami and Jose, the only other male nurse, the nurses were all sensitive, sweet-natured, caring women. The doctors on the other hand, including Dr. Wunder and the entourage of residents who followed him on rounds every day, were all very Alpha male, leader of the pack, hetero-type manly men. From my perspective, it was interesting to observe having so many female and feminist friends. Could there actually be something to those stereotypes of the nurturing, gentle woman and the dominant, hunter/killer man?

In addition to the doctors' rounds, the vital signs, pills, and twice-a-day dressing changes were the defining features of my days. Routines were stacked upon routines. The nurse opened this little, prepackaged, sterile tray of supplies. They ensured they never touched anything and cleaned along the incisions with sterile saline solution. An antiseptic gel-covered webbing called Bactigras was placed over the skin graft to prevent the gauze from sticking to anything. Then came the gauze, thick protective padding, and lots of tape. The remains of the kit were thrown away. This happened twice a day. A part of me was horrified to be the cause of such ecological waste, but, if it helped me heal safely and hastened the process in any way, I was okay with it. Little did I know.

The day after I switched to the Zimmer splint, I was visited by my inpatient physiotherapist, Andrea Browne. With the help of Stephen, a big, burly bear of a man, I was hoisted out of bed and placed in a chair with the call button near my hand. The world spun, and a wave of nausea overcame me as I sat upright for the first time after being horizontal for five days. I was actually able to sit up for a half hour, stubbornly enduring until the dizziness faded. By the time I was returned to bed, I was exhausted.

The next day, I was helped from bed and placed in a tall, wheeled walker with a padded collar and handles. I stood in the walker's embrace with my arms along the padding, gripping the handles with all of my limited strength. With Andrea on one side and Stephen on the other, I made it to the door of the room while hopping on my good leg. When he came by on his daily rounds, Dr. Wunder said my jaunt had put me ahead of 90 percent of the people in my position. To me, every success was a failure. I always wanted to be further along, to be better. I had not yet learned to scale back my goals to something achievable. The new yardstick I would have to use to measure my life and accomplishments hadn't arrived yet.

The following day, I graduated to a regular walker and made it out the door and about twenty feet to the nearest intersection of corridors. After that, my training with crutches began, even though I wasn't allowed to use them alone for several more days. Around the room, I was allowed to get up and, using the walker, go to the bathroom again.

The return of even this minor bit of mobility did wonders for my spirit. I could bathe myself in the bathroom sink and use the toilet, even though I mostly used the little plastic bottle to urinate and the routine of bathing was enough to tire me out for hours. I was also able to forgo the hospital gown and wear shorts and T-shirts. Because of the scarlet red dressing over my graft donor site, I could only wear loose shorts. Boxer shorts were collected. I received a blue-and-green plaid pair from Pauline and several pairs from Kerry. Dressed even this casually, I began feeling vaguely human again.

The second weekend after the surgery, drainage was still coming from the edges of the skin graft. One of the Wunderettes took swabs along those edges and sent them to the lab. The news wasn't good.

◆   ◆   ◆

06*0?*00

I've lost track. I have no idea what day it is. All I know is it's Sunday.

I've developed some infection along the upper and lower sutured edge of the skin graft, and I'm terrified. I'm floundering, and I don't know what the parameters of this are. How bad is this?

I have terrifying visions of them having to redo the skin graft that set my pulse racing.

I wept today—often. I didn't even care that my hospital roommate could hear me. Once the tears ended, I just wanted to sleep. I actually fell asleep listening to Bach for a while despite the endless nattering in Spanish of the family sitting outside the door.

Gods, I just want to go home. I just want my own bed. I feel exhausted and yet the whole battle of healing is still ahead. But I guess the worst is over. The cancer is gone, but the road back is a long one.

◆   ◆   ◆

As I fell into despair over the news of the infection, I heard Dr. Wunder talking in the hall. I don't know who he was talking to or about, but I heard him talking about a young woman somewhere down the hall who wasn't going to live. Suddenly, despite the intensity of my feelings, I felt very lucky to be alive. However, two diametrically opposed emotional states wrenched me.

On Monday afternoon, a team of doctors from infectious disease control visited. The woman in charge poked and prodded while discussing me with her team. There were no outward signs of a systemic infection. There was no unusual amount of pain. My temperature and blood pressure were normal. I felt fine, or I at least felt as fine as I could under the circumstances. A new course of IV antibiotics was prescribed: Tobromycin once a day and Meropenim three times a day.

I think I surprised her when I asked for the worst-case scenario. She looked at me and said, "You don't really want to know that, do you?" I was quite vehement that I did. I think I showed admirable restraint by not freaking out when she told me. Inside, the ground fell away.

◆　　◆　　◆

06*0?*00

Well, I definitely have an infection, pseudomonas. Apparently, it is a bad, fairly resistant strain. The infectious disease specialist doctor says, from the looks of it, the fact it's in two different spots means that it seems to be superficial. We'll just hold onto that because the other possibility is that it's inside and coming out. In that case, they have to take the prosthesis out, clean out the infection, and put the prosthesis back in again.

Oh, fuck.

I'm running out of strength. I can't take anymore hits. I just want to be healing. I just want to know that it's actually getting better. Will this never end?

◆　　◆　　◆

That was the last thing I wrote in my cancer journal. There are just blank pages after that. I don't know why. Maybe I was just too tired, too worn out from the fight. Maybe it was just my procrastination or my well-known habit of rarely finishing what I start. Maybe I felt my cancer was really over; that part of the journey completed. Maybe that last one is just what I'd like to be true. I don't know.

Any subsequent scraps of thought I had were written in either a school subject notebook or a little, red, bound, two-dollar book I carried around in my bag. There were many thoughts to write down…because the journey was nowhere near complete.

Ten
The Road Home

If the infection the doctors detected in my leg had indeed been systemic and if it had indeed invaded deep into the healing mass of tissue that was my new knee, the results would have been severe. They would have had to go in again, reverse all they had done, and remove the prosthesis until the infection cleared up. Without any joint, my leg would have just been left without any structure to hold it straight and very little to hold it together. I would have had to undergo the reimplantation of the prosthesis and more reconstruction. It was another horrifying prospect bringing on another tide of fear. In the days that followed, the diagnosis of the infection and the lines of the incision above and below the graft began turning sullen red. However, my vital signs remained normal. No signs of a deep, systemic infection appeared.

Linda visited every day. We'd talk, and she'd knit. She would bring wool and a pattern for knitted washcloths, saying she needed something to keep her occupied, that is, to keep her from fretting. She finished several of them before she even arrived.

After her first ride on the subway, she announced she didn't like it. The sensation of travelling without visual references to indicate movement bothered her. As far as I know, on every trip to and from the hospital, she took the streetcar along Queen, but she always walked the distance between Queen Street and the hospital.

I'm ashamed to admit the one instance when I snapped, when my anger and frustration at what was being asked of me and what I was enduring, was at Linda. I don't remember the catalyst. It could have been in those first few days of having seen the raw wound on my leg, when I felt so ugly and completely maimed. Maybe it was when I had gone a few feet down the hall in my walker and returned to bed, shaking with exhaustion and cursing myself for not accomplishing more. Whatever the cause, I was feeling on edge and beaten down. My emotions were rubbed raw. When she said something about how much worse it could have been, my control broke. Through breaking tears, I commented, "That's easy to say if you're not going through it."

The hurt on her face went through me like a kick in the balls. Whatever I felt disappeared, and what remained was deep sorrow for opening my mouth. I started crying and tried telling her how sorry I was. Her eyes were wet as she told me it was all right. Then she went outside for a cigarette. When she came back (in true King family tradition), we didn't speak of it again.

Gordon's play, *The Watch for Sunrise*, the play that had taken so much of his energy and time for the last few months, received its reading on June 2. I was still in the hospital, having only come out of surgery the previous week.

I was devastated I couldn't be there. We had talked about his experiences with the playwright's circle, and I had seen the passion he held for this piece and the amount of work he had put into it. And now, when the piece was making its debut, I couldn't be there.

It touched a deep well of guilt. I had taken up writing much later than Gordon, but, once we were both involved in the craft to our respective extents, we always exchanged work. When I stumbled through my first novel, he was the first to get a copy. He paged through it all and gave me extensive notes, never anything that would crush my spirit or make me stop, but he never let me off if something didn't ring true or if I was overdoing it. He even developed his own acronyms for my recurring flaws. RA was redundant adjective, and TUT was tells us twice. The same thing happened with each successive project. He did the same thing, sending me various versions of his projects. I read them when I could, but, more often than not, they went into the black hole that is my life, ending up on a shelf or in one of the piles of paper that characterized my living spaces for so long. He would ask if I'd read them. With a shrug I'd say something about my latest crisis or lack of organization. He would just take it in stride and never stopped giving me his latest material. I was doing it again, missing something that had meant so much to him.

As I write this, I realize how little I've actually talked about him in these pages. I suppose it gives the impression that he wasn't that great a part of my life during this time. Nothing could be further from the truth. We talked about it at some point during our discussions for this book. What he did for me during those months of radiation and waiting that was so precious was just be normal. The frequency of our visits didn't change. We weren't always together. We talked on the phone, and he always let me talk about what I wanted to talk about. I was always just Stephen, never Stephen with cancer. He didn't freak out to me. I never had to deal with his traumas, fears, or issues. After the surgery, he dubbed the scarlet red dressing over my skin graft my "Scarlet O'Hara." He was the one to bring long, slim rainbow stickers from a shop on Church Street to run along my crutches like rally stripes. To me, he was a rock. Any upset he might have had was thankfully offstage. On some days, it seems like I have known him forever.

◆   ◆   ◆

My antibiotic schedule kicked into full swing as soon as the infectious disease team saw me. I had my dose of Tobramycin every morning; a dose of Meropenim followed. The other doses of Meropenim followed at eight-hour intervals. At those times, I was bed-bound and hooked to my IV pole. The morning doses took the longest because the Tobramycin had the potential to eat away at my veins if given too quickly. It had to be administered slowly.

Once I was unhooked from the IV, I had a small amount of time when I could move around. While I was learning to use the crutches, I wasn't allowed to move around with them alone. But each morning, with the walker, I was allowed to go to and from the bathroom and sponge bath in the sink. Using either my other foot or a grip extender, I could get a clean pair of shorts over my leg and shimmy them up over the Zimmer splint. It was a little taste of freedom after the days of bedpans and urine bottles, a taste I was anxious to maintain. Of course, the simple act of washing and changing my clothes left me so tired that I needed to lie down again.

I continued my lessons on the crutches with Andrea, going a little farther each time. Eventually, she taught me the proper way to take stairs, using a three-riser ministair that led nowhere. Once she was certain I could manage an entire flight of stairs without hurting myself, thus allowing me to get in and out of my second-floor apartment, she would proclaim me fit to return home…after the infection cleared.

I was also wheeled down to the fifth floor, bed and all, where they did an ultrasound on my leg and found no evidence of blood clots, which was more good news. After a few days of rotating saline locks on my arms, I was taken for the next little stage of my medical journey. The nurses explained what was going to happen.

Because I was to be on antibiotics for six weeks after getting out of the hospital, instead of rotating the locks in my arms (I would have looked like a pincushion when I was done), they were going to implant a PIC line in my arm. The line would be inserted through my arm into a vein and guided through my body to a point near my heart. The advantage to this procedure is it can remain there and be stable for a long period. It sounded horrifying, the thought of this "thing" so deep inside me. But there was no choice, not with weeks of antibiotics ahead.

I was sent to the X-ray department for the insertion. On the table, my left arm was stretched out. I was given a needle full of anaesthetic, which, again, hurt like a son of a bitch. Then a needle was inserted into my bicep. A guide followed, which was positioned as they watched it on the X-ray. Positioned along the guide, a small, slick, silicone tube followed along the veins through my arm and into my chest. Other than the pain of the anaesthetic needle, the only sensation I felt was when they were sidetracked in the wrong direction into a smaller blood vessel. It didn't hurt. It was just an awareness of the line's presence, somewhere near my shoulder.

The procedure was over in less than a half hour. It was an odd feeling, even more Borg-like, to see this valve that extended from the skin of my bicep and know the tube extended deep into my body. I eventually got used to it. It was just another of the strange sensations and strange experiences that were piling up daily.

The days passed. They watched for signs of deeper infection, but none arose. One day, as Linda was having a cigarette outside, she met a woman named Carole, whose daughter, Julie, was in a room down the hall. Julie was undergoing chemotherapy for an osteosarcoma in her shoulder. Linda and Carole became buddies as they went for smokes outside the hospital. (They were smoking while helping family members with cancer. Don't even get me started on that little logic loop.) Carole often came down the hall for a visit. She and Julie became inextricably bound with that time in my life, and, as you will see, would return later.

I was immensely proud of Linda then. Despite being emotionally wound up from supporting me, she found the time and energy to make a friend and be there for her. She and Carole still e-mail back and forth to this day. That's what it's all about, isn't it? Taking the time out from whatever trials and life shit we're going through to lend a hand to someone who needs a bit of help. I found a lot of that in the cancer community, people who, despite the crushing burdens of illness, have moments to spare for a smile or kind word and provide a small moment of connection in the face of the juggernaut. Whenever possible, I still try to do it as well.

Before I was released, Linda had to return to Saskatoon. If my original timetable had been adhered to, I would have been home before she had to leave, but the arrival of the infection sent that timetable flying. I was still days from release when she had to leave. We said good-bye in my room, hugging fiercely. Gordon was there and followed her down to the lobby just to ensure she was all right. She went back to the apartment, finished her packing, and caught a car to the airport.

I missed my family deeply through all of this. I often wondered if it would have been easier if they been close enough to drop by the hospital during visiting hours. I suppose it would have been easier for me. I wonder if it would have been easier for them as well, instead of having it all happen so far away.

Dave, from the next bed, was the next to go. Despite having his surgery after mine, he was up and around and discharged while I waited. Exchanging e-mail addresses and phone numbers, we said our good-byes. Once more, I was swept up in my longing to be out of that room and that bed.

A new roommate moved into the room, but there was no great bond this time. He was just an extra in this little drama with no lines written in the script. More days passed, and home care was arranged for my eventual departure. Several times, I asked when my release would come. The date kept getting pushed back. I got my strength back in small amounts. I mastered my crutches.

Then, three weeks to the day after my surgery, the day finally came. I didn't actually see Dr. Wunder; just a Wunderette. He gave me prescriptions for Percocet and signed the papers. It was that simple. Pauline came, and we packed up the cards, CDs, books, and magazines I had accumulated. We dismantled the almost-home away from home. With my leg nice and secure in my Zimmer, we slowly made our way to the elevators and the lobby. After a brief stop and wait while my prescription was filled, we called a taxi. I dropped into a seat as we waited, being tired from the sheer effort of moving in a crowd of people.

When the taxi arrived, we were presented with the monumental task of levering me into the back seat. Using the trick I had actually been using before the surgery when my leg had been so sore (lifting the limb by putting the other leg under it), I could slide back along the seat with my legs up. It was awkward, but the feel of the sun on my face and the breath of even Toronto air through the open window was sheer heaven. Maybe it was just that I'd been trapped inside for so long. The sky was that paralyzing shade of blue that's only seen on clear summer days. From my reclined position on the backseat, my perspective was skewed. (I'd get used to it because it was the only way I could get to and from appointments at the hospital.) All of the buildings seemed impossibly tall, like I was looking through a child's eyes again, a good metaphor for the process I would go through in the next months. It didn't matter. Only one thing mattered. I was out.

Eleven
Home

On that clear summer day, when the cab pulled up to the house, Pauline took my bag like a Sherpa guide. I hauled myself out of the backseat. I pulled myself up the three concrete steps to the front porch, using the technique Andrea had taught me. Place one crutch on the side opposite the handrail, and hold the other crutch in the hand that's around the handgrip of the supporting crutch. Lift yourself to the next step by placing your weight on the handrail and the one crutch. Repeat as necessary. Enter through the downstairs door and then the apartment door. I went one flight of stairs (miles long on that first day), and I was home. I was so winded that I went straight to bed.

There was no time for a nap though. (I've never been much for taking naps anyway. Naps always leave me feeling dazed and sluggish.) Boxes of medical supplies were already on the living room floor. Baggies of antibiotics were chilling in the fridge, awaiting my return and the arrival of my home care nurse.

Around two o'clock, my traditional time of medication, Sandra Polsky arrived. Unlike the nurses at the hospital, she was dressed in casual street clothes. There were no bland, pastel uniforms here. She had dark, chin-length hair. Within minutes, I could tell she had sass. I've never liked people who tell me what I want to hear. Unless I've explicitly told you that I want my sensibilities indulged, I would rather be told the truth, whether I'll like it or not. I knew right away that I could count on Sandra for this. She never let me indulge my self-pity, kept me grounded when my spirit started flagging, and felt free to razz me whenever she felt so inclined. I mouthed off to her often, and she gave it right back to me. Deep down, I respected and liked her. (She eventually called herself Nurse Ratched.) Perversely, with me, it's a sign of respect if I give you a hard time. It says I think you've got guts and a good soul. Don't ask where it came from. I don't know.

That first afternoon, she took my vital signs, set up the loops of IV tubing from the IV pole that became a fixture of my living room for the next few months, and gave me my first dose of Meropenim. We discussed the when and how of my care. She said she just wasn't going to come at six in the morning. Eight o'clock would be just fine. I was okay with that. I gave her a set of keys. Pauline was still in school then and was often gone during the day. I couldn't negotiate the stairs every time someone rang the bell. After a few days of rest, I decided to go on the balcony and drop keys at whoever was visiting so they could let themselves in. It seemed silly to do that with Sandra because she would be in and out twice a day. So, with a gift of a set of keys on a key ring shaped like a shark, our relationship began.

The first few days were spent negotiating my way around my home. Once taken for granted, it was now a threatening maze of unfamiliar space. I quickly realized my relationship to it had completely changed. The knowledge this change had affected my whole life and world, not just my home, would come later. The landing along the main stairs, leading from the bathroom and kitchen in the back, past my room to the living room and deck in front, suddenly seemed precipitously narrow with my new aluminum appendages. Narrowing the spread of the crutches along that confined piece of floor decreased my stability. During those early days, I always felt like I was going to topple over the railing into the stairwell.

Everything in those days was logistics—how to get to and from the bathroom, how to arrange myself on the toilet in a narrow bathroom with a leg that sticks straight out, how to make food for myself, and deciding where to eat it because I couldn't carry anything from room to room. (Anything that could be gripped in the same hands that gripped the crutches was okay. Coffee mugs and plates of food were impossible. If I wanted to eat, I did it in the kitchen.) I also had to figure out how to get in and out of bed, how to get on and up from the sofa, and how to bend down to reach the VCR. All these day-to-day actions I took for granted had to be pondered, analysed, and thought out. I often had to wait and make sure someone else was in the house in case I fell or injured myself in some way. In the end, I simply adjusted and found ways to do things or came to terms with the fact that, for the moment, I couldn't do them.

My days quickly settled into another routine. I was up just before eight o'clock, usually having gotten out of bed and onto the couch when Sandra arrived. My old habit of watching *Whose Line Is It Anyway?* first thing in the morning, set when I lived with David and Trish, reasserted itself. It would play in the background as Sandra disposed of the previous days IV tubing and strung up a fresh set, including a fresh bag of saline. I warmed the first bag of antibiotics under my arm. She would hang it lower than the saline and let it drip. Gravity makes the drug go from the bag into your arm. Whatever is hung lower on the pole drips in first.

The procedure for this became burned in my memory, and I soon learned to do it myself. First, the valve end of the PIC line had to be wiped with an alcohol swab and then flushed with 10 cc of saline solution. Then, the IV was hooked up, and the drip rate was adjusted. After the drug was finished, the saline must drip for a few minutes to flush the line. There was another 10 cc of saline; 5 cc of Heparin followed. Each flush required a disposable syringe.

While the antibiotics were running, Sandra changed the dressing on my leg using the same procedure as in the hospital, except without any dressing kit. Each day, a set of plastic forceps were placed in a cup of water, covered with plastic wrap, and placed in the microwave for seven minutes to sterilize them. In the box of supplies were dozens of individually wrapped gauze pads, Bactigras sheets, and cushioned absorbent pads. For the first week or two, we changed the dressing twice a day.

Each day, we threw out plastic tubing, an empty saline bag, four empty antibiotic bags, nine syringes, two old dressings, and the wrappings for all the elements of the new dressings. I was a one-man ecological disaster.

After *Whose Line*, we watched a home decorating show with a host we nicknamed "Blinkie" because of her disconcerting habit of completing her entire introduction without blinking once. After filling out my chart, Sandra left and returned around one o'clock or two o'clock in the afternoon. If Pauline was home, she made coffee and sat with us. If Pauline was gone, I had to make coffee for myself and drink it in the kitchen.

My mornings were spent watching an hour of stand-up comics on the Comedy Network. It then watched often-seen repeats of *Star Trek* while I read the paper and did the crossword puzzle. After that, I checked out Donny and Marie. If there were no interesting guests, I had my sponge bath. I stood in my bathroom naked and propped against the sink with all my weight on the good leg. With a sink full of water and one of the washcloths Linda had knitted, I washed as best I could and then got dressed.

The thing no one tells you about sponge baths is that you never feel properly cleaned. You don't feel disgusting or smelly, but I had no idea how much I missed that "fresh from the shower or tub" feeling.

By the time I dressed and wrestled together something for lunch, I was ready for a rest. I was usually back on the couch by the time Sandra returned. Once my afternoon dose was over, I either read or watched more TV. After I was more confident on my feet, I made it to the balcony to sit and watch the world go by and feel the sun on my face.

After dinner, (again, I ate in the kitchen if Pauline wasn't home to carry my meal into the living room), I watched more TV until the night nurse came in for my last dose and evening dressing change. After the news at ten o'clock, I went to bed. This was my routine for weeks.

The Sunday after I returned home, with Pauline at my doddering side, I made it down the stairs, out of the house, and all the way to the corner. I don't know if you've ever been on crutches, but, with only one weight-bearing leg, you are reduced to this sort of swinging motion. Both of your legs are straight, and all of your weight is on the good leg. It takes a lot of effort to hoist your body weight forward. I needed five or ten minutes on a bench at the corner before I had the strength to return home. I lay down for a while once I levered myself back up the stairs.

During our visits, I learned Sandra was as much of a reader as I was. She lent me the first three Harry Potter books. I lent her Katherine Neville's *The Eight* and Diane Duane's *So You Want to be a Wizard?* We talked about all kinds of things, including my feelings about my situation and our mutual love of our neighbourhood. Sandra was also a fan of the Tango Palace, my favourite neighbourhood café. I truly enjoyed her company, as I did the others who came in the evenings or on the weekends. There was no-nonsense Camellia; sweet, soft-spoken Marissa; tall, dark Sal; and Raquel, who looked barely old enough to be out of high school. I treasured the company of these caring women because I was often alone during those days. With Kerry gone and Pauline completely immersed in schoolwork, I was often alone in the house for hours at a time during the day. For me, conversation was often as curative as the antibiotic.

Gordon came over frequently, bringing crossword books and a huge pan of pasticcio that he cut up and froze for me. When Pride Day came, I desperately wanted to go. The parade has always thrilled me since I've been here. I love the spectacle, the happy energy that courses through the crowd, and the joy on the faces of the participants. Sandra put her foot down and said there was no way I could brave the crowds. Gordon and David joined Pauline and me for pizza and cocktails on the deck. We then watched the first episode of the British *Queer as Folk* on video. You should have seen me trying to get down the hall on crutches after having my first drink of alcohol in more than a month.

One night, Gordon and David came over and made nachos. I ended up especially glad for their presence because Kerry came by with Ken to pack up some stuff. It was the first time Ken and I met, and it didn't go well. Kerry proceeded to pack all of his CDs, including ones we had bought together, into boxes. He said, if there was anything I wanted, we could sort it out later. I was still too shell-shocked and exhausted to do my happy dance to make everyone else feel comfortable. Thinking I was just opening my mouth to make a joke, I made some comment about him taking them all now so he could have them all without me putting up a fight. It came out bitchier than I intended, and he responded in kind. The bitter wars were on again. When I realized what I had done, I just stopped talking to avoid any escalation. Ken just stood there uncomfortably. Gordon seethed at Kerry for picking that moment to pack. After they left, he asked when the tone of sharpness between us was ever going to go away. I said I didn't know.

He asked if it was maybe time to distance myself from Kerry and the relationship. I said I couldn't. I needed him. When Gordon asked why, I didn't know how to answer. The only things that came to mind were concretes, such as having someone get things for me and running errands I couldn't do. I think now I know I just needed any link to my past and the normalcy (or what passed for it anyway) of my former life. The life before cancer and the prosthesis destroyed the world that I knew, the world that was safe.

Gordon took a more active role in those postsurgical days. He brought vitamin E oil and pure aloe vera gel to help minimize my scars. When *X-Men* opened (an event I had been waiting for all year and an event, even in the hospital, I swore I was not going to miss), Gordon came with me, shepherding me on my first foray on the streetcar. (I had already been on a bus once with Pauline to drop off the paperwork for my disability claim at the Employment Insurance office. We actually got the driver to lower the hydraulics and drop the floor of the bus for easier access.) We shared the movie in a warm, comic lover's dream come true sort of way and dissected it over coffee afterward.

When I had to begin my routine of postsurgical follow-up appointments at the hospital, Gordon accompanied me. He held the crutches as I stretched into and out of the backseat of the cab. He followed me through the soaring glass atrium of Princess Margaret to the sarcoma clinic. He was there with me on June 27 when the staples were removed. He held my hand, as I gripped his fingers like a vise as the stubborn ones were pried out. (Because of the healing complications from the radiation, the staples were left in longer than normal to ensure the incisions and graft had truly healed. Some staples had healed or scabbed over.) He pushed me to breathe when the searing pain made me rigid. Looking at him through tears and feeling like a total sissy, I said, "Well, that wasn't very brave, was it?" He just put his arms around me and said, "Sometimes you just can't be brave," and handed me a tissue.

Twelve
Emotional Roller Coaster

When I returned home from the hospital, I had an e-mail from Michael, the great kisser with the unhappy relationship. He was just getting in touch and wondering when I'd be home. I called his number. In a notable change from the last time I called, the message had only his name on it and a forwarding number if people wanted to reach the boyfriend. It seemed I wasn't the only one going through changes.

I left a message to let him know I had finally been released from the hospital. I didn't ask about the boyfriend, figuring he would tell me if he wanted. We arranged for him to stop by and visit.

When Michael showed up at my door, I hobbled to the balcony and dropped the keys. He was wearing long, but well-fitting, black, jean shorts and a loose, muscle shirt. Both suited him quite well. His skin was dark and well-tanned. Later, he said it was just the way he was. On the other hand, I, because I missed nearly the entire summer and was a pasty British boy, was fish-belly white.

We had a nice visit. He said his boyfriend moved out the weekend before he came to see me at the hospital. He had still been in shock when he saw me. He hadn't felt it was appropriate to tell me, considering what I had just been through. We talked, and I confided a little of my feelings about the scar and the deep well of insecurity about my attractiveness. I must confess, with his new-found singleness evident and the underlying spark between us twitching to life, I flirted a bit. I employed those gentle touches. I placed my hand on his forearm and brushed my knee against his and left it there. I didn't push too hard, but there's something nice about touching. I don't mean groping, kissing, or anything heavy like that, just pleasant human contact. Once you've French-kissed someone and you find you actually like them as a person, it's silly to maintain a wall of distance between you.

When it was time for him to leave, I broached the subject of the lingering attraction I could tell was still there. He agreed, but we both knew we weren't really in any position to do anything about it. So we agreed to leave it and just spend time together.

Meanwhile, I got some strength back and began venturing out on my own. I made it to the end of the block, across the street, and around the corner to a little bakery I love. While I rested, I had a butter tart and fizzy lemonade. It was the beginning of my freedom to move about on my own, and I treasured it. I just watched the world go by on sun-drenched Queen Street East. Each time I went out, I slowly pushed my wanderings a bit further. One day, I even managed to get myself on the streetcar, travelling only as far as Broadview to get a coffee. But I did it myself, and I conquered a big fear in the process. Each day and with every journey, I pushed myself harder and to do it better while battling the fatigue and limitations.

With my crutches and the Zimmer splint in plain view, my disability was quite obvious. Most people were quick to jump up and offer a seat. I always found it delightfully ironic that the first person to offer was usually in the one seat that would put my stiff, straight leg right in the path of everyone getting on or off the streetcar. But people were kind. They often asked how I was and what had happened to me. It was odd. I told them I had my knee replaced, but I hesitated saying the "c" word. I always felt somewhat self-indulgent telling people I had cancer. It smacked to me of some kind of grand, "pity me" ploy. I think it also had something to do with the shocked looks on their faces. Cancer is still a big bogeyman. There are still many gothic horror notions about the disease, and some are completely justified. But I've noticed the change in how people look at you when you tell them you have cancer.

My walks culminated in actually being able to make it all the way down Queen to the Tango Palace. I had to sit for a good rest afterward, but I did it. I think those days were marked by a desire to confront my limitations face on. When Sandra told me I should get out more, I promptly went further than she thought I should. As soon as I was able to do something, I did it. As I got more confident in my ability to move around, my state of mind definitely improved.

◆   ◆   ◆

07*24*00

Tonight was a night for medical programming on TLC. Michael told me about a show on the hospital where he works, St Michael's. Curious to get a feel for the place, I watched.

Well, they managed to hit all of the buttons. Orthopaedics, cancer, and knees. Before I knew it, the submerged emotions (time bombs as my friend, Sandra calls them) were surfacing. Next thing I know, I'm crying streams of tears and wracking sobs. Like a car wreck, I wanted to tear my eyes away, but I can't.

The program tracked back to a young woman who was hit by a car. A strip of skin had been torn away from her left knee. (Not only was it the same body part, but it was the same side.) The narrator talked about how they had to call a plastic surgeon and do a skin graft, taking skin from her hip. A feeling rose in me, and I thought, "Oh, that poor girl. That must just be awful." I then stopped and realized how similar it was to what just happened to me. Suddenly, I was howling with laughter. Tears of hysterical laughter replaced my tears of grief and shock. It's funny the power we have to disassociate ourselves from our own trauma.

My sister Linda began a raffle at her job for a coworker whose son has osteosarcoma and might lose a leg. She came up with the idea to raffle an afghan she knitted. When she told our mum about it, Mum said she would give a couple of paintings to add to the prize stash. Linda told her she didn't have to do that. Mum responded, "Well, you never know when it's going to happen to you." There was a pause. "Oh, that's right. It did happen to us."

At least I know I come by it honestly.

◆   ◆   ◆

Another visit from Margot further buoyed my spirits. She had been in Ottawa over Canada Day to sing in a thousand-voice choir, another event I wanted to attend that was now denied to me. She could swing through and stay a few days with us. It was a wonderfully low-key visit. My strongest memories are two-fold—good and bad.

The base of my left foot was dry and scaly because there was not any sock or shoe or pressure on the sole. I often sat on the couch and rubbed my other foot against it, creating a shower of dead skin cells. Margot sat with me one night, ever so gently peeling away the dead cells. She then rubbed lotion deep into my foot. It was such a small thing, yet it was like cutting my toenails, an act I couldn't accomplish myself. It needed to be done, yet it seemed so intensely personal that I hesitated to ask. Poor Pauline got to do the toenails a couple times, as did Kerry.

My other memory of Margot's visit is a painful one. We were watching TV when a Reba McEntire video came on. (Why do that woman's videos push buttons?) It was about being a rock for someone you love and always being there. I wanted Margot to see it, to tell her in some clumsy way that I appreciated her

being there for me all these years and I would always be there for her. I only managed to make her cry. The video changes from a woman being there for her
daughter to the daughter caring for the mother when she becomes ill. Margot lost
her mother and father in short succession. She looked at me with tears in her eyes
and said, "No sick mommy songs!" I would gladly have been swallowed up by the
earth at that moment. But, like the friends we had been for most of our adult
lives, she forgave me. Nothing active. It was just a slip back into the comfortable,
old ways. I never brought it up again. I couldn't face even a trace of that look in
her eyes again.

I continued recovering. Very soon after starting the round of antibiotics, Sandra
and my evening nurse, Sal, showed me how to hook up the IV and run the drugs
myself. The evening visit was discontinued after a couple of weeks. We arranged for
me to handle the afternoon dose myself if I wanted to go out somewhere.

I was on these fresh tastes of independence like a shark on blood in the water.
I took every opportunity to shake away my dependence on other people. I hated
needing people for things like my toenails or helping me put on sandals. (I did
like the homemakers they sent to do my laundry and clean the bathroom.) I
loved being able to free myself even a little from the routine of the drug doses. I
had a love/hate relationship with being cared for. I had always been independent,
and my life since my diagnosis and surgery had revolved around the things I
needed from people. With surgery severely limiting my mobility, my need for
care suddenly grew exponentially. I constantly bridled at needing someone for
anything. With the small doses of increased independence, I began feeling a bit
more like myself, maybe even a little better than before.

◆   ◆   ◆

07*??*00

There is something new in my face when I look in the mirror, some new set in my eyes.
Arrogant as this sounds, I find myself handsome consistently. Before, I often had days
when I actually saw glimpses of the handsomeness that people have told me is there.
But they often faded quickly, chased away by ugly duckling memories of childhood.
Then, all I saw was the fat, out of it, faggot outsider who was tormented for so long.

Now though, it's different. When I look in the mirror, I see something else. I see my
features, good ones. Nice eyes. Nice lips. Good bones. Maybe it's the weight I've lost.
I've lost more than twenty pounds since moving here. Regular weigh-ins at the clinic

prove it. Divorce and cancer burned away the pad of fat. All of the planes of my face are exposed.

But it's more than that. It's something deeper. The changes don't stop at the skin. My soul has changed. I guess it's stronger. Maybe, like it burned away the excess fat, the cancer burned away a layer of doubt or uncertainty in my own strength, revealing the steel beneath.

Odd. I look at the scars on my leg. Though they are healing well, I can only see them as ugly. My leg has been marked in a hideous, extensive way. I can live with it though. It is part of me. There is no going back or getting away from it. That ugliness has saved my leg, if not my life, but it will never be anything besides a jagged flaw.

Yet, strangely, ugliness of my leg seems to have made my face more beautiful. My friend, Mike St. Denis, told me of a friend of his who had open-heart surgery and now wears her scar proudly. He said she told him that she now understands the difference between merely pretty and truly beautiful. I think maybe now I do, too.

◆   ◆   ◆

Of course, it was never that simple. On many days after writing this passage, I still felt brutally damaged and haunted by the spectre of the fear that I was flawed so deeply that no one could ever love me again. The battle was not so easily won. One day, I realized, after I had been moving around reasonably well on my own for a while, panhandlers didn't hit me up for change anymore. I guess they felt sorry for me. It was a blow to my healing and confidence. I mean, if street people feel pity for you, your life is really fucked.

Michael and I talked almost daily, having conversations that ranged from our families to circumcision and everything in between. It became a habit that we would be in touch before bed every night. One time, he came over, and we shared a bottle of wine and pizza. I told Sandra I was having a date. I think, without our actually declaring it as such, it was.

It was nice to just sit and talk while occasionally holding hands. I think gay men shortchange themselves in the area of dating. Our sexual politics sometimes seem to dictate a hurried leap to bed. The political line seems to be that we aren't like those nasty heterosexuals, so we don't have to model their behaviour. I know this isn't true of everybody, so don't write angry letters. I just found, in my own life, I was so anxious to have the validation of being with someone that I tumbled headlong into relationships without stopping to just spend time with the person. I saw Kerry go through it as well in his search for someone after we split up.

Michael's recent split and my healing body prevented us from rushing into anything. Or so I thought.

While talking one night and sharing our nightly lullaby of words, he said something about having gone to the bar with friends and not having the slightest desire to meet anyone. He said the reason was he felt like he was already dating me.

It was music to my ears. My fears about never being desired again melted away. No, that's not right. They flew away as if they were jet-propelled. At the time, I couldn't see that, even though I really liked Michael and desired him sexually, I was mostly just earthshakingly glad that someone felt that for me as well. The ugliness of my leg wasn't going to be an issue. I mean, he was a nurse, right? He would have seen things in the ICU that would have curled my hair, if I still had any. Surely he wouldn't be put off by a scar, regardless of how large.

◆   ◆   ◆

07*25*00

There are days when white-hot, seething anger comes upon me from deep inside, morphing from magma to lava. The most recent occasion was the week of my mother's eightieth birthday. The initial plan was to surprise her with a barbecue in Moose Jaw. My sister in Saskatoon would drive down. My niece Pam would come from Winnipeg with her basset, Henry. All was in place. The hitch came when they found out my cousin Karen and her husband Russell were bringing their new baby through Saskatoon that very weekend. As well, Karen's parents, my dad's sister Gill and her husband Roger, were going to be there as well. It was a fortuitous complication, but it was a monkey wrench in the works. Plans were quickly changed, and the surprise became Pam's arrival.

I was here, laid up on my couch with a padded brace on my scarred, rebuilt leg and a line leading from my arm to an IV pole. See the dictionary under "pissed." It was possible I could have travelled with a steamer trunk filled with supplies, of course, and someone to change my dressing for me. But there was no money.

I got angry. Once the rage came, so came the checklist of things this has taken from me.

Let's start with my knee. Can't get much more concrete than that! The complex set of bones that make up the joint has been sawed out of me. (I've seen orthopaedic surgery on TV. It is hard, grunting work like something out of Bob Vila or the Furniture Guys. Knee replacement by Ed and Joe.) A hinge made of metal is now jammed in its place and immobilized for three months until the bones grow into it.

We can add to the list a self-image, a body consciousness shattered by two-and-a-half feet of scar down my leg. (I was getting closer to the real length, but I was not quite right yet.) *A lumpy, twisted mass of rearranged muscle and grafted skin is on the side of my knee. It's ugly. It's mine, and I honour the fight it represents. However, it will never be anything except ugly to me.*

If we want to talk about occasions missed, let's talk about Pride Day. For the last two years, the parade has been important to me, a symbol of my new life here. (The year before, I had gone despite being half-dead on my feet with a flu bug. I just propped myself up against a building to wait for Gordon to come from work and let it all pass by me in a blur.) *This year, it is a chore to get to the bathroom. I had barely mastered cooking for myself. Braving the crowds of millions on the street? Out of the question.*

The list goes on. Rogue cells pulled events, emotions, and situations from my grasp. (This included Gordon's play, Margot's performance in Ottawa, time away from a job I loved and people who were a joy to work with, and even something as simple as going dancing, which was something that had filled me with joy in my Saskatoon, pre-Kerry days. I remember the swell of pride I felt when Kim, a girl who took her dancing very seriously, looked at me and said I was one of her top ten favourite people on a dance floor. That was gone, too.)

This almost cost me my burgeoning relationship with Michael, but we were both wise enough to realize there was something here worth pursuing if we went very carefully. That's one less thing to be angry about. Perhaps it's a Karmic blessing or gift from the gods as repayment, if you believe in those things.

◆   ◆   ◆

At the time, I wilfully blinded myself to the fact that Michael and I did much better on the phone than in person. His manner was always awkward when we were together, a stiffness that went through his body when I got close to him. Even after we decided we were dating, it was nearly two weeks before we were actually in each other's presence at a barbecue at his apartment.

He said he wanted me to come over to meet some of his friends. He also said I could stay over. When the day came, I backed up my knapsack with a toothbrush and some clean underwear. Michael came and got me. I tried fitting in the front seat, but the Zimmer held my leg too straight. It was the backseat for me again.

At his place, he gave me the tour and made dinner. I started seeing bits of the discomfort he felt in my presence. He flitted around the kitchen, not stopping too close to me very often. Then he showed me pictures of his ex. That should have been a big clue.

Dinner was lovely. I met his friends. We talked, ate, and laughed. After his friends left and it was just the two of us, just as the Rubicon was about to be crossed, we faltered.

Poor Michael. He just wasn't ready to be with anyone. His breakup had really knocked him for a loop. We sat across the kitchen table from each other, and he just looked miserable. I felt it as well, but I didn't want to blame him or make it anymore difficult. He was a decent man who made me feel good again. He just wasn't ready. Truth be told, in hindsight, neither was I. He offered me the guest room, but I asked him to take me home. As he drove, apologising at least twice more, I reached forward and squeezed his shoulder. Even with the way things had turned out, the warmth of a touch was comforting. It was just as much for me as I hoped it was for him.

I couldn't be angry with him. The memories of the shattering grief and confusion I had felt when Kerry and I split were too fresh in my mind.

I went into a tailspin for several days after that, but it wasn't really because of the failed attempt at a relationship. It was because I had done again what I had done so many times in the past. I attached too fast. This time, I placed all of my desires to be loved again and to feel attractive and good about myself on Michael. I didn't blame him in the least, but, to my trauma-addled mind, it was my last chance for a relationship. I had felt I couldn't be desired, and this just proved it. That was my fault, not his.

Weeks passed that I was locked in proximity to my IV pole. More routine…more repetition…more medications…more dressing changes…more visits from Sandra. On July 26, I took my last dose of antibiotics. The six weeks were finally over!

Within days, I developed vertigo. For the following two weeks, every time I moved my head, the room spun, leaving me queasy. I started moving very carefully on my crutches. I discussed it with Sandra, and she continued checking on me. My next follow-up appointment was only a couple of weeks or so after the antibiotics ended, so she told me to bring it up with the doctor.

My friend Jen visited in early August, passing through town on her way to Montreal for a summer class. She's an intellectual property lawyer in Edmonton. On the surface, she's petite, blonde, and girly, but she's sharp and tough underneath. She and her boyfriend of many years, Travis, were mainstays in my McKim Apartment days in Saskatoon. It was a joy to see her. Travis's presence was the only thing that would have made it better. I missed them both fiercely, as much as I missed my family. If you want to know the truth, I really think of them as family, my family of choice. I think my years in the McKim were the happiest of my life. I had dear friends all around me, and I felt stable and content in a way I haven't achieved since. After I left, the group began scattering. Even if I wanted to go back, it's actually a state of being I'd want to go back to, not the physical place. That state is a thing of the past, but seeing Jen again was a warm reminder of that time in my life

Those few days were fun. Jen took some pictures of the apartment and us with her digital camera. We took a walk through the neighbourhood, ending up at Tango Palace for desserts. The day was only marred when Kerry opened his mouth about how uncomfortable I had made Ken the night they were over. He'd already pissed me off by teasing me about my studly love life in front of a woman we knew while we were in one of the nearby stores. I was still stinging from the Michael thing and did not have any patience for it. The veiled accusation about Ken was too much. I stopped talking because I didn't have any energy to deal with it.

On Sunday, Kerry took Jen to the Royal Ontario Museum I admit I felt resentful because he commandeered part of her time with me. In many ways, while we were together, my friends became *our* friends. When he made new friends after our split, he didn't want to share them. None of his friends I had met tried staying in contact with me, but he expected my friends to stay friends with him. Jen, however, made it all right when she answered my strong yet immature desire about wanting to know that my friends liked me best. She simply smiled beatifically and said, "No, we *love* you best." (When asked if he would stay in contact with Kerry if I somehow stopped speaking to him, Gordon, bless his heart, answered tactfully, yet clear as thunder. "It wouldn't be a priority.")

The Tuesday following Jen's departure, August 8, was an eventful one. I had to go for my three-month X-rays of my leg and lungs. One of the things they must monitor is the appearance of spots in my lungs. If this cancer was going to spread anywhere, that's where it would be. For the first year, I had to have my lungs checked every three months. Then, it would be every six months. Then, it would be every year.

When I was on the table, the X-ray technician asked how big the prosthesis was. I had to admit that I did not have any idea. She took her first images, and I heard her disembodied voice say, "Man, that's big!"

After the X-rays (which were clear), I had my follow-up appointment. Dr. Wunder wasn't all that concerned about the dizziness, and it passed after another week or so. He was quite happy with my progress. He wrote me a prescription for physiotherapy at my last appointment, and my first session was that afternoon. Perhaps the best thing that happened that day was the removal of the PIC line. Another in the unending line of Wunderettes simply placed a gauze pad over it and pulled. Out it came, and I didn't feel a thing. But the symbolism was clear. The antibiotics were over.

That afternoon, I met the woman who would guide me through the next phase of my recovery, Joanne Beasley. Joanne is tall and willowy with chin-length, curly hair. She initially seemed reserved, and it made complete sense when I later found out she was originally from England. She emigrated with her family when she was ten or eleven. I knew it all too well.

That first day, she looked at my leg and measured the degree of bend I was capable of. That day, it was fifteen degrees. She immediately started me on my program. She put a towel under my left thigh and told me to grasp the ends, pull up to lift the leg, and make the knee bend. After a half hour, she attached me to a biofeedback machine with the electrodes placed on what remained of my quadriceps. My task was to clench the muscle to make it register on the machine to increase my mind-body connection. Then she took the leg and bent it by using brute strength. The pain was unbelievable and seared right to the marrow.

I saw her twice more that week and every day the following week. The week after that, it was every day. And every day the week after that. Each session took two hours. She told me to think of it as my new full-time job.

I met the woman Joanne jobshared with, Dawn Rodie, a sweet, soft-spoken woman with a policeman for a husband and a daughter just under two years old. I soon learned the differences in style between the two of them. Joanne seemed tougher on the surface and was more willing to push me harder. Dawn, on the other hand, was shorter and quieter. She seemed to be gentler, but, now that I think about it, she managed to push me hard as well.

I went to the hospital every day. Every day, I went and endured pain like I had never felt before. It was the only hope I had for getting off the crutches and walking again.

So much of cancer treatment consists of routines, steps that must be executed repeatedly. These steps have no efficacy in the individual, only in the cumulative effect. Radiation…antibiotics…physiotherapy. My life during the months of dealing with this disease was all about these mind-numbing patterns.

◆   ◆   ◆

08*10*00

The crazies (the mood, not the type of person) visit me all the time now. I'm tempted to charge them rent. Since Michael said he wasn't ready for dating yet (just an instigator, not a real trauma), the floodgates are open. I feel broken inside with all sorts of sharp edges rubbing against each other.

I broke a closed thermos once and heard the shattered metal lining rattling around in my chocolate milk. I feel like that these days. I have to cover a huge distance before I can walk or sit normally again, not feel the shattering pain when Joanne bends my leg, or simply have a leg again. It will be a scarred, ugly leg, but it will be a leg and not a dead lump of flesh.

Thirteen
Physiotherapy

The incisions were almost completely healed. The only thing that remained was a small bit of persistent drainage from the folds of scar tissue at the top of the skin graft. There wasn't a dressing anymore, just a sterile gauze pad I could change myself. Sandra was coming only once or twice a week now, and the physiotherapy gym consumed my world.

Every day, either at ten o'clock in the morning or one o'clock in the afternoon, I reported for my appointment. I had graduated from the towel under my thigh to a pulley and strap contraption that provided greater return for my effort. Plus, it was a good workout for my arms. After a half hour, I did another half hour on the biofeedback machine. Then Joanne or Dawn sat and patiently manipulated my kneecap from side to side, attempting to work it free of the adhesions and scar tissue from the surgery.

By this point, Dr. Wunder had given me the go-ahead to begin bearing weight. Joanne tested me by having me place one foot on each of two scales. By shifting my weight back and forth over the scales, we could tell how much weight I could bear on the bad leg. From the first try, I could bear nearly 120 pounds of weight on the healing leg without pain. The bending was proving to be a challenge.

Joanne settled on a new routine to help with the bend. I sat on one of the pneumatic beds with the foot pedal that controlled the bed's height at hand. Sitting over the edge of the bed with my foot resting on a stool, I raised the bed until the knee bent. We later added weight to my ankle to push the process even further.

Each visit always culminated in either Joanne or Dawn holding my leg and using sheer force to make the knee bend further. It was almost three months before the brutal pain lessened even slightly.

I met some lovely people during my times there. Judy, a sweet, older, Jewish lady, had broken a bone in her arm and was trying to get it back into shape. She was on the bed next to mine and in obvious pain. She once asked her therapist, Anne, how many more she had to do. From my bed, I piped, "Ninety-two!" Judy threw back her head and roared with laughter. We were pals after that. Every time she came in and I was there, she told Anne, "I have to say hello to my boyfriend."

Robin, a nice lesbian, just wanted to play hockey again. Jennifer, tall and dark with Whoopi Goldberg hair, had broken a bone in her leg while riding a motorcycle.

It's funny. One day, I thought how much fun we often had in the gym despite the fact we were all enduring pain. Regardless of our respective injuries, our pain seemed to bring us together. We were always laughing or teasing each other.

Even the staff was a joy to see. They were all friendly and supportive. I knew, even if I was having a shitty day, I'd come around the corner and Lucy, the receptionist with big hair, big heels, and big smile, would always bring a smile to my face. Kind people were at every turn on my daily journey to and from my appointments. Patricia, the sweet girl from Argentina, worked at the hot dog stand outside the hospital. I had developed the habit of stopping for a veggie dog after my sessions, and Patricia always gave me this huge, dimpled smile and asked how my leg was that day. Eventually, I began receiving a big hug along with the smile.

The sweet, round-faced Indian woman worked at the newsstand in Queen's Park subway station. On one of my many stops there, she asked what had happened. After I told her, she always gave me a big smile as I passed.

Even Joanne's initial reserve melted. She and Dawn looked out for me emotionally and physically. They knew how hard I was working better than I did, and they saw how hard I was on myself and how much emotional strain I was under. Joanne suggested seeing a psychiatrist who worked with cancer patients. She talked to Dr. Wunder about the referral, sending me into Dr. Jon Hunter's care.

Joanne said she and others who had dealt with him all agreed he was the most normal psychiatrist they had ever met. For me, he was one of the easiest people to talk to. I felt safe with him, safer than I had felt in months. At our first session, he sat scrunched up in his chair with his feet on the table. There was something so natural and honest about him that I knew I wanted to stay in his care, despite time constraints that only allowed us to meet once a month. When I told Dr. Satok about seeing Dr. Hunter, he said he continued to feel I was in the best hands because he had worked with Jon at the beginning of his own career.

Inside, I think I knew the care I was receiving was top-notch. Despite the pain I felt during those times and the frustration at how slow things seemed to be moving, I always felt as if there was a point to it. Among those people, there was safety and help in that place. They would get me though this.

◆   ◆   ◆

I don't feel connected to my body anymore. After six months of this disease and its treatment, thirty-seven years of being in this flesh doesn't matter anymore.

◆   ◆   ◆

During the second week of my physiotherapy, on August 16, my parents arrived. They had arranged a visit to make sure I was all right and to take care of me for a while.

It's amazing how, even at my age, there is comfort in one's mommy and daddy. As soon as they arrived, I felt somewhat like a child again, desperately craving to be held and rocked to sleep and have my way eased. But the old patterns of British reserve fell into place. I didn't want them to see the trauma and pain. I didn't want to put them through even a taste of what I had experienced. I can only imagine how it must have been for them, that is, to be so far away when their only son was going through cancer treatment and extensive surgery. I couldn't let them see the dark side.

My mother cooked and made enough meals to last for a couple weeks after they went home. My father puttered around the house, fixing this and that. At one point, he went to find a model train store. As with every other visitor that summer, we went on the ritual ROM visit. I even took them around the hospital. They met Joanne and some of the nurses who had taken care of me during my stay. (Whenever I was in the hospital for physiotherapy, I always stopped by the ward to see if anyone I knew was there. They always seemed glad to see me and were genuinely pleased that I was doing well.) When I took them by the radiation unit, my mother started crying and wandered off down the hallway to try keeping it from us. Shannon was such an angel. She put an arm around her and offered a tissue. Mum could only manage to quietly say, "Suddenly, it's all real." When Shannon took us in to show them the machine and explain how it worked, Mum was fine again.

The week they were here was comforting. We fell into those safe, old patterns of having tea and watching the news and Britcoms on TV. It was nice to be taken care of.

When the day came for them to leave, my mother wouldn't let me come downstairs. She didn't want me to see her upset. So I waved good-bye from the balcony. The day they left was August 24, three months to the day since the surgery.

◆   ◆   ◆

It is the three-month anniversary of my surgery, and it should be somehow marked. What were the events of my day?

I had my first shower in three months. It's the first time I've felt clean in that time. I washed and scrubbed my back twice, once with soap and once with an alpha hydroxy scrub to try to clear away the zits erupting on my back. The one spot at the edge of my skin graft that's been draining (it finally stopped scabbing over on the weekend) lost the scab in the shower and began oozing again. After three months, it still hasn't healed.

I sent my parents home today. After they left, I had such mixed feelings. It was wonderful to see them, but it was tiring to play the stoic, stiff upper lip routine. They didn't want to see the pain, fear, frightening loss of control and dignity, and the loss of self-esteem from being scarred so profoundly. Mum cooked meals, and Dad fixed things around the apartment. Pep talks were liberally interspersed.

I'm so fucking sick of pep talks and people telling me how well I'm doing and how much better the scar looks and how nobody will ever notice. I just want someone to respect my pain and loss and all the gut-wrenching trauma.

Physio continues. Every day for at least two hours, it culminates in blistering pain as Joanne or Dawn bends the knee. There are gains measured in millimetres and degrees of bend that fade to nothing overnight. It's a long, slow, torturous process that leaves me weak.

I just want to feel concrete, observable progress. Healing. I don't want anymore yellow gunk from scabby, unhealed parts of the incisions. I want movement in the knee that I can keep from day to day. I want something other than a baby step.

I checked my diary tonight. My first appointment with Dr. Taylor was in January. So, even if you discount Peter's initial opinion at that first checkup, this has been happening all year. It has been eight months and counting, and there is no end in sight.

◆   ◆   ◆

When your body is as profoundly changed as mine was and when your healing process requires you to get around on crutches for three months to avoid putting weight on one of your legs, your relationship with the world is thrown into disarray. Your physical relationship to the space your body occupies is suddenly nothing like it was before. There is no way you can relate to the world in the same ways that were once completely familiar. Your perception of space changes, but the way people treat you changes as well.

This became doubly evident when Joanne made me stop wearing the Zimmer splint, except when travelling on public transit. When I was walking around, my leg and its scars were exposed. I became acutely aware of the way people looked. Yet, I tried so desperately to act as if they weren't looking. The scrutiny was intense, the feeling I was under a microscope. I could practically hear the thoughts, "Oh, that poor guy," or "What happened?"

I pushed myself. I could have just worn long pants, but I refused. The thought of being exposed like that terrified me, so, in true, stubborn, Aries Stephen fashion, I wore my shorts and didn't let the fear stop me.

During that time, I met a man. I walked around a corner, and there he was. From that first second, I thought he was very sexy, but my gaydar said nothing. We exchanged pleasantries and went our way.

I was lucky enough to run into him again. This time, I threw caution to the wind and gave him my card. Coincidentally, we were travelling in the same direction on the streetcar, so we had chatted until we reached my stop.

We talked on the phone a few days later and decided to have lunch. It's funny because we sat through the meal and I still had no idea if he was even gay. I told Joanne the following week that I might have had a date, but I wasn't sure. I didn't know for days until we were sitting at my place one evening and he leaned over and kissed me. That settled that.

It's difficult to write about him because he's firmly in the closet. Not one person in his life besides me knows he's gay. To this day, I can't believe I could have fallen for someone who wasn't out. I think, if I had known initially, I might have steered clear. But, at the time, he made me feel safe. I felt a peace in his arms that had not been a part of my life for months, if not years.

I don't know. I maybe just needed someone in that difficult time. I even tried telling him that. I tried making him see that I was still an emotional wreck in many ways. He said he understood, but he wanted to try anyway.

The closet thing was an issue that cropped up repeatedly in the time we were together. I gave up playing those games a long time ago, and I think, if I was in a position for a long-term, emotional partnership, I would demand it of my partner. But I felt good with him, and there were so many other issues I needed to sort out. So I just took the comfort, pleasure, and love where I found it. I needed that feeling because, just below my determined surface, I was so completely unnerved and unsure of everything I was and had once been.

He was an anodyne to that. On some level, I perhaps used him, but I tried my best to be as honest as I could about emotions that I was only just getting a handle on.

I practised at the gym constantly, taking multiple tours around the room. I moved ungainly on two canes. Day after day, I focussed on the "bend, step, lock the prosthesis, shift weight" pattern that would be my new gait. Joanne taught me how I would have to climb or descend stairs from now on. Unable to bear weight on the altered leg unless the knee was straight and the prosthesis locked, I would only be able to lift with my good leg. For the rest of my life, I would climb stairs that way and descend them by lowering my weight onto the good leg as well. Eventually, I was given the go-ahead to use one crutch. After a couple weeks, the day came when I could make the transition from crutch to cane. When I walked into the Tango Palace to meet Gordon for the first time after making the switch, I will never forget the joy on his face as he watched me from the pay phone in the back.

◆   ◆   ◆

09*18*00

_____ *called me his little hero. Yesterday, Gordon told me this is the stuff of heroism. Is it?*

I don't know. When you're in it, you're so preoccupied with the struggle as well as the pain and drugs to control it. There is fatigue from dragging your body around on crutches. There is weakness from the dregs of the general anaesthetics that can remain in your system for a year. There are hours of screaming exercises that are designed to help you walk again.

Even the moment when I put aside my crutches for the cane (a moment that made those on my support team misty with tears of joy to see it) felt less like a triumph and more like a relief. Just being able to walk without needing to rest every few blocks is a release.

So many of these small triumphs are swallowed in the day-to-day living with some-thing like this. They are lost, along with so much, in a personal neurosis of feeling like I'd be further along in my recovery if I was just a bit stronger or a bit better at coping with the pain.

Heroism? I don't feel qualified to comment. It's hard to feel like a hero when you need someone to tie your shoes for you.

◆   ◆   ◆

I talked to Joanne about that feeling of that nagging doubt that the lack of progress in bending was somehow my fault. I was getting stronger. What remained of my quadriceps was strengthening daily. But the ability to bend my knee normally continued eluding me. I began feeling like I was letting the team down. She was quick to remind me that I was working hard, but a part of me didn't believe it.

I was seeing Dr. Hunter, the psychiatrist, by then. He was a refreshing, safe place to go in order to deal with all of the shit that comes from dealing with cancer. He asked why I was so ready to give credit to all of the doctors, nurses, and friends for all of their hard work and not acknowledge my own. I didn't have an answer.

When I expressed the thought that I should not give in to the doubts, fears, sadness, and strain, in typical Jon fashion, he said, "Well, here's the thing about positivity. It doesn't work. Studies have been completed. What matters more than a constant sunny outlook and really helps people recover faster and better is authenticity. Being honest about the feelings you experience and the effects of your struggles serves you better than blind optimism." This was good to hear. For the most part, I have been the type to know if I am feeling pain, sadness, or some other dark emotion. It is a place I pass through, and it is not a place I take up residence. I usually know I will feel better in the morning or in the next few days. Jon told me it's a Buddhist concept called mindfulness. Perhaps its the equivalent of "This too shall pass."

While I was struggling with my feelings, both for _____ and my own lack of progress, the world continued turning. At the beginning of September, Kerry officially moved out. The months of squabbling, confusion, and nonrelationship were finally over. I was too tired and in too much pain to really mourn its passing. I think I'm glad of that in a strange way. My grief at the end of a long, serious relationship was just bundled in with all of the other pain and began healing without any undue fanfare. It was just another part of the whole experience. An old friend and former roommate of mine from Saskatoon, Dave, moved in, so the change occurred with a minimum of fuss. There was nothing I could do anyway. I was in no position to help anyone move anything, so I just stood back and watched it happen. I then continued on my stumbling way.

◆　　　◆　　　◆

09*19*00

On some days, it's exciting, this journey of rediscovery. When we are children, our journey is to make sense of the input from our new senses, to collate all of the chaotic sensory input. We learn as we grow to navigate the world, to connect to it and find our place in it. We learn the uses and limits of our bodies.

It's kind of like this. At thirty-seven, my relationship to the world and even my own body has suddenly changed. I have to rediscover all of these relationships. Nothing is the same. Because my leg won't bend properly yet, I can't sit, stand, walk, bathe, or move in the ways I used to.

Using crutches or a cane means never going anywhere without needing a resting place for objects. I need something to hook them on to free my hands or something to lean them against. Not only that, I need something to lean them against in such a way that they don't topple to the floor (because it's not an easy thing to bend down and pick them up).

I can't hurry. It's a physiological impossibility now. My gait is slow. If I'm imprecise in how I put my foot down or lock my knee between steps, I run the risk of falling.

There are patches along the back of my leg I can't feel anymore. My relationship with long pants has changed. The numbness feels strange against the material.

My big toe on my left foot no longer works. It's a minor thing really, but it's disconcerting when any part of your body doesn't work anymore. Plus, as it points slightly downward, it can catch on the edge of carpets or things on the floor. That can force the knee to bend suddenly or beyond its capability. And that can hurt.

◆   ◆   ◆

One day, I came home and found a hard dose of perspective in my e-mail.

◆   ◆   ◆

TO: stephen
FROM: linda
SUBJ: News

Got this at work this morning. I should respond, but can't think of a goddamned thing to say. I'll figure it out eventually, but not today. Everyone here is a little distracted today because this is the day Sam Clarke (remember, the son of Ken, whom I work with) has his surgery. The doctors have decided to do rotationplasty. You should look this up on the Net. It's much easier to read than for me to explain.
Talk to you soon
Lin

from: Carole
To: linda
Subject: News

Hey Linda,

Well, I got to see Stephen when we were in Toronto last week. It was good to see him doing so well! I did see him another time, but he didn't see me. I avoided him because I just couldn't deal with things. The bottom line we got while there is that they sent us home because they can't do anything else for Julie. They actually recommended we stop all treatments and just let her go. Now you know why I couldn't face Stephen a second time. Needless to say, we're shocked, angry, devastated etc....

So, we're back home. We're lying to everyone because she doesn't want anyone to know, planning lots of trips, and talking with the oncologist here to see about other options. They told us that they can't operate on her lungs. There are too many spots in nonoperable areas, and they'd have to amputate her arm from the collarbone down. (There is no point if they can't do the lungs.)

So, it sure was hard saying good-bye to everyone there and coming home to pretend that we're just going to transfer her treatments closer to home then take another look in a few months.

Sometimes, it's so hard to just make it through the day pretending that everything is normal. She goes back to see the oncologist here this week, a great guy who firmly believes we can't and won't give up yet. I see my doctor tomorrow to talk to him about other options.

Julie went into full shock when we were told, but she has decided not to deal with it right now. So, she's actually the stronger of the three of us. She's out with her friends as much as she can.

Anyways, that's what's happening here. Feel free to pass it on to Stephen, but please don't let it go any further. (It is a small world, and we don't want it coming back somehow.)

I'm thinking about you a lot. I miss our friendship and hope things continue to go well for both of you!
Love,
Carole

◆   ◆   ◆

I'm at a loss. I can't sleep. Grief is thudding in my ears, so I do the only thing I can. I write.

I found out a young girl who was in the hospital at the same time as me, a girl of eighteen, not even out of high school, is dying. She has an osteosarcoma in her shoulder with metastases in her lungs. To amputate her arm, they would have to take it off at the collarbone, which is pointless because the spots on her lungs are in too many inoperable places. So they send her home to die.

My first impulse is to give her the rest of the time I have been granted if it was only possible. I've been alive twice as long as she. I've had a life full of blessings. I've acted and learned. I've loved and lost, written novels, and shared the joys and sorrows of many a dear friend. Knowing _____, I have known love even at a time of great stress and difficulty. There are things I haven't gotten to yet, but many other blissful surprises that have taken their place. Let her have my turn. She deserves it.

At the same time, I know what a specious, empty sentiment it is. No matter how sincere I may be, my conviction can never be tested. There's no magical sci-fi machine to make the switch. My fate is mine, and hers is hers.

I wonder how I can ever face Carole again. How she could ever look at me and know I survived the fate that has taken (will take) her daughter's life? How could she ever feel anything but hate for everything I represent?

I was feeling amazing today—full of hope and luck. I felt joy at being alive and healing. Now those things are still there, but they are shaded with a more somber appreciation of how lucky I really am. As every day goes by, I realize just how big a bullet I dodged.

◆   ◆   ◆

I've had a day to process the news about Julie. Mostly now, I just feel lucky to be alive and healthy and doing well in the face of all of this.

Underneath it, in a corner of my heart, I no longer have the luxury of ignoring. I feel shame—deep, burning shame that I have been granted this precious gift of life and health when this beautiful child is going to die. What great, cruel cosmic imbalance gives me my life and takes hers?

Why does it persist? This insane notion that the universe is somehow a fair place and virtues are rewarded and vices punished by a just, cosmic order.

You would think, after twenty years of HIV and AIDS, that this silly notion would have been burned out of me for good, cauterized like an old wound from my psyche. But there it is again.

◆   ◆   ◆

I talked about this with Dr. Hunter. His only real comment was about how powerful survivor's guilt is. It's true.

The years of my early adulthood were the years of AIDS. I was no angel. I used sex (and sometimes anonymous sex) as a balm for my insecurities, loneliness, and feeling of never belonging. I was careful, but I didn't feel I had been that careful. I don't know why I was spared. When Tom died and then Frank and Glen, I couldn't help but wonder, "Why them? Why not me?"

At one point in my chequered youth, I indulged in a threesome. The other two men are now dead. It took years to reach some kind of peace with my life and realize it wasn't something I had or had not done. It was a virus, and viruses don't discriminate.

Now I was back there again, and the survivor's guilt was rushing over me once more. How could I go on, knowing Julie was going to die and I was going to live? What had I done to deserve this great boon? The news touched the deep insecurities that I didn't deserve to survive and what I had done with my life was not worthy.

Of course, there aren't any answers. Cancer is just cells. Like viruses, cells don't discriminate. All you can do is go on and know that some clichés are clichés for a reason. There, but for the grace of God...

Fourteen
Peaks and Valleys

There's a tree across the street from my house, sitting at the edge of the school's parking lot, that signals autumn every year. I never notice a gradual change in the leaves. I just look out one day and see the tree has turned gold and red. For the last few years, the temperature drops suddenly, like someone has turned off summer with a switch.

◆　　◆　　◆

09*22*00

On some days, it's hard to remember that you're lucky to be alive. On those days, the boundaries of your world are pain to the north, south, east, and west. On those days, you struggle to lift your foot, and sharp knives go through the bones you have left. You then repeat the motion over and over for a half hour. On those days, you hang there with your foot dangling off the edge of an elevating bed, reaching the limits of your bend. And your foot just hangs there.

On those days, the pain overwhelms you. You sit in a room full of people weeping, trying desperately to conceal it (proper British repression always asserts itself), but you can't even speak, lest the floodgates burst.

All you want is relief, a moment or two without your body protesting the hoops it must jump through, just to get you functioning in some approximation of normalcy.

On those days, it's hard to remember that each day you wake up is a gift.

◆　　◆　　◆

Like any other person in any other life, there were good days and bad days. I began growing accustomed to my new, modified body, even though the end of my journey would be a long time coming. It wasn't really a conscious process

108

most of the time. You simply get up each day and your new limitations are still there. There are minute variations, but the overall picture remains the same.

The sun rises and sets. You get up and travel into the world in your new mode, your new physicality. And you just slowly get used to it.

My physiotherapy continued every day. I went for dinner with ___. We grew more comfortable with each other, but, like I have always done, I often felt the urge to flee. I used to go to a tarot reader in Saskatoon named Phoenix. She was a blast to spend time with. Even on the days when she was totally inaccurate, I looked forward to seeing her. In a flash of insight one day, she said I tend to see the potential in others instead of the reality. As a result, I usually end up disappointed. She has been proven right so many times, most often in my romances. I've let my illusions and my senses of the person's potential blind me to the realities and the requirements of making relationships work. With ___, I wanted to make sure, if it came to an end, it wouldn't happen because I bolted prematurely. I was never sure if my feelings were just a symptom of the disease and recovery. I told him how uncertain I was about everything in my life. I was just vamping until the long recuperation was over.

When I felt overwhelmed by the sheer weight of what had happened and what was still happening, he held me while I cried.

◆　　　◆　　　◆

09*27*00

I just realized I've grown quite accustomed to my scar. I was bothered when the weather turned colder, and I had to wear pants. I was happy today when it turned out to be nice.

I'm sure it's subversive on some level. I like scaring people or confronting them. I guess I always have. It doesn't get much more in your face than this.

On some levels, I think of it as a quest to reeducate people, that is, break down the walls of beauty and perfection stereotypes that bind us all. We can all be beautiful, even if we don't fit the norm.

There's also an element of it being a badge of honour. With all I've been through, I've earned this mark. It's a reminder of my survival, of beating the cancer and surviving the ordeal.

I guess I also like the occasional bit of special treatment it affords me. I always get a seat on the streetcar.

Damnit, I'm beautiful and it's part of me, so it's beautiful too.

I went to see Gordon at PJ's on Saturday and overestimated how cold it was. I could easily have worn shorts. I joked with him that I could have been in my shorts scaring people. Imagine it, walking through the ranks of perfection-obsessed homos in the ghetto with an eighteen-inch scar down my leg. It would have been like Moses parting the Red Sea, or John Hurt in the Elephant Man. "I am not an animal. I am a human being!"

Nothing subversive there. Nunh-uh.

◆   ◆   ◆

I read this now, and it sounds so insufferable. Reeducating people? As if my scar has the power to change the world. It was another step on the road to just feeling comfortable in my own skin again, but it sounds unbearably pretentious now.

I think I must have sounded a bit like that when I met Mike Forbes. I continued to stop by the ward where I had spent my weeks after the surgery. Jane always gave me a great big hug whenever I saw her. One day, she asked if I would mind meeting one of her patients, who was actually in the room I had occupied. She wouldn't tell me about his diagnosis. She just said he was gay and thought I might be able to help him. Well, in my newfound desire to remake the world, that was music to my ears.

Mike was a nice, young man from Winnipeg. He was there to treat osteosarcoma in his ankle. I met him and his boyfriend, Skip, and the other man in the room. The tumour in Mike's ankle had gone completely through the bone. The night after I met him, they amputated his leg below the knee.

I stopped by to see him over the next few days, gave him my card, and said, "If there's anything I can do, just call," several times. I put on the grand survivor mask and acted like the elder statesman of cancer, the wise sage who has all the answers.

Mike actually seemed to be fine and coping quite well. The day after surgery, he was moving around on crutches. I remember feeling ripped off after the days and weeks of my struggle to get upright again. I actually thought, "If amputation was that easy to get over, why hadn't they just cut off my leg?" (Joanne later said that mid-thigh amputations are subject to more serious complications.)

When I said good-bye to Mike on the day he flew home, he sounded grateful we had met. I don't really know if I did him any good, but we still keep in touch.

I now realize just how deeply he touched in me a powerful desire to help in some way, to give back some of the good fortune I had received.

◆   ◆   ◆

This terror comes over me sometimes, pouring over me in waves. I don't even know what I'm afraid of or where it comes from.

I went shopping today. I had to meet Kerry and give him some mail. While I was out, I found some things I wanted—some funky fridge magnets with quotes on them and a book by Judd Winick about his relationship with and the death of his friend and Real World castmate, Pedro Zamora.

It hit me like a ton of bricks. I wept like a child at the friendship and the loss of another bright light. I guess I'm just susceptible to illness stories these days.

These terrors lurk under every stone, waiting to jump at me. I don't even know what I'm afraid of. Dying? Maybe. Pain? Definitely. The thought of a recurrence of the cancer terrifies me because I probably know just how bad it could be if my lungs were affected.

No, these fears are too specific. This is more a generalized thing. It hovers like a cloud at the edge of your vision. Then you find yourself thinking of your new boyfriend, job, or your friends. Suddenly, the cloud is over your head, casting a bleak shadow over everything. Suddenly, you're scared you've imposed on your friends' good nature too much. Alternatively, you see all of the potentially relationship-crashing differences between you and your new boyfriend and begin dreading an end that isn't even in sight. And you just want to hide under your bed.

◆   ◆   ◆

Judd Winick's book hit me so hard because of the empathy I felt for him as he watched Pedro sicken and die. Did my friends and family go through that? We had never really discussed it. I was too busy with my disease and recovery to stop and wonder about their pain and fear. They were too busy helping me by being strong and supportive. Was it horrific for them to see me go through the surgery? Did they wonder in the dark if I was going to live? Do they now catch themselves wondering if they would have to shepherd me through this again?

How could I allay their fears when I couldn't do anything about my own? Or could I?

◆   ◆   ◆

10*03*00

I had an epiphany this morning while waiting for the streetcar to come to physio. In our world of Calvin Klein model, six-pack, buff-bod, Barbie perfection, where we are bombarded every day with images of how physically perfect we could be if we just worked out a bit more or ate a bit less (or had enough surgery), I'm suddenly free.

With my scar and the obvious physical flaw, it has become impossible for me to be perfect. I can't exercise it away, smooth it over with alpha hydroxy or anything like that.

I can be strong. I can be beautiful. I can be fit. I can be buff (granted not likely, but possible). But I can never be perfect.

It's quite freeing. Suddenly, my body can be a testament to the truth we should all believe, but so rarely do. One doesn't have to be physically perfect to be beautiful.

Not to make myself sound saintly or any such twaddle like that, but I think it's why I'm happy to wear my shorts. (What a change that is!) It's an act of—I don't know—defiance, maybe? Maybe it's just a small act to show that it's okay to be different and physical imperfections don't stand in the way of beauty and happiness.

◆   ◆   ◆

10*03*00
P.S

The Lord giveth, and the Lord taketh away.

Today, Joanne said, despite my work, she doesn't think I'll ever get ninety degrees of bend. It's not a matter of hard work or pain tolerance; it's just the physical limits of my flesh.

I felt like someone had kicked me in the gut. I didn't actually think I'd had any expectations as to how well I'd eventually be. I guess I did.

Of course, my forebrain said all the right things, "I just want to do as well as I can and I just want to be able to maintain it."

But in reality, it's pretty devastating to know the best I can hope for is to be some-
what less handicapped than I am now. I will never have my normal function back. I
guess I always knew it, but I always hoped.
Fuck. Fuckety-fuck. Fuck-a-doodle-doo.
____ of course says it doesn't matter. We'll get through it together.

◆   ◆   ◆

I struggled to absorb the news. The radiation had damaged my tissues in its
mindless assault on my cancer. Like skin suffering from bad sunburn, the elastic-
ity was gone. However, in my case, the sunburn went completely through my leg.
The prosthesis was capable of ninety degrees of bend, but the flesh it was set into
was not.

There is a deep shift in your perceptions when you realize you are handicapped and your inhibited mobility and function are permanent. There is no "all
better" to look forward to. But you do what you have to do. You add it to the
weight you carry on your shoulders through life, shifting the balance of the load
until you become used to it.

The week before Thanksgiving, my sister Jennifer visited. For years, I har-
boured the secret feeling that she had never forgiven me for being born and
usurping her place as the baby of the family. But we've actually become friends in
the last five years or so. Though she was the last to find out I was gay, she took
Kerry to her heart and made him feel welcome in the family. When she met
____, she did the same. She even cooked me an old-fashioned Thanksgiving tur-
key, something just out of reach of my culinary skills.

She had always been the cool one. I remember talking with her on the phone
one night during my radiation treatments, and she said how she just wasn't worried because she felt everything would be all right. But she cried when I took her
by the hospital.

◆   ◆   ◆

10*14*00

I'm sitting in the Chapters at John and Richmond, holding a Mocha Frappuccino in
hand. I had to stand on the streetcar almost the whole way. (Damn the cold weather.
With my scar covered up, I was just another young, healthy-looking man. There goes
the sympathy factor!)

Being among the bookshelves again, I want to go back to work so badly. My disability is running out. I'm becoming scared about whether I can go back or not. I can't stand or sit for long periods. What am I going to do? Do they even want me back?

Long-term disability is an option if the insurance company will pay it, but I'd rather be useful somewhere.

I feel at a loss. There are so many things I could be doing with my time—the memoir, learning to type better, or reading. Yet, there's this malaise. I don't know where to go from here and what I'm capable of anymore.

◆   ◆   ◆

10*20*00

I'm overwhelmed. My feelings burn, making my eyes sting with tears. I've reached fifty degrees of bend. I howled, but I got there. Joanne says it's amazing, that it's where she wanted to get to. She also says it's probably the best we'll get. Pushing me through burning hell, she might get ten degrees more, but, in her opinion, the law of diminishing returns kicks in.

There may be improvement in the future from day-to-day living, but this is the best we'll get through this process. She says I've come a huge way and should be proud of myself.

I am. My spirit soars at having beaten the odds and getting the best I can, of having made a goal and not giving in. Yet, there is sorrow as well. Grief wells at the final loss of the rest of my mobility, the final death knell of normalcy. I must let it go now—my former able self, my dancing and long walks, my speed of movement, and my ability to run from trouble. I can't stop the tears now. The sobs wrack me, and the saltiness tracks my cheeks. There is so much joy, grief, and intense everything. Stress, pain, fear, love, and hope pour through me.

How much easier it would all be if emotions were discrete, separate things and if we could feel one and only one, without messy overlap and without the smearing mess of them running together.

Now comes a spike of thermonuclear rage. How dare the fates do this to me? How much can one man take?

More tears. I sit outside the hospital with the pigeons and the traffic. I shouldn't be angry at fate. I was lucky, but the pain has been so hard. I feel like my back is breaking. I can feel the crunching of my bones as they snap under the load.

But I'm still here. There's no sudden blackness. The pigeons still fly and peck at seed on the concrete. The cars still stream by. And I must go on. I must work at this for the rest of my life, or I will lose what I have gained, what I have worked so hard for. And I won't do that.

◆   ◆   ◆

The day after I wrote that, Gordon and David got married on a lovely Saturday afternoon.

_____ came with me. It was our first social gathering as a couple. In the church after the ceremony, Gordon and I held each other and wept. At the reception, I was a witness and signed the marriage certificate and register. It was an honour. _____ and I sat at our table among friends, and he put his arm around me. I went to bed that night feeling warm and happy, but I woke up feeling sick.

It's something that happens to me. Being so good at repressing my feelings, I can hoard them until the stress makes me physically ill and I have to just stop everything for a day or so to get my bearings. _____ seemed to think I was mourning the final end to my long-gone relationship with Gordon, who had been my first love so many years ago. It hadn't occurred to me, but I don't think that was it. I'd laid that ghost to rest a long time ago. I was overjoyed to see my dear friend marry the man he loved. It was just that, coming on top of my emotional train wreck of Friday, the wedding was overwhelming. In the light of their happiness, I was still broken and disabled. The bipolar pull of grief and joy on me were too much, like I was being torn in two. I just had to catch my breath.

There's only so much a body can take.

◆   ◆   ◆

10*24*00

I had a really bad case of "Why bother?" today, combined with a burst of rage that left me weeping in the washroom down the hall from the gym.

Sobbing, I thought, "Is this it? Is this what I've worked so hard for? To be Peg Leg Pete who can't cut his own toenails? Who needs to be accommodated at work? Who will always have a leg that sticks out and is in the way?"

I talked a bit with Joanne about it all. Her husband wrecked both his legs in a racing accident so badly that they would have amputated them if he hadn't refused. (I guess I got off pretty easy.) You just have to lower your benchmarks of what success is.

Success for me is walking reasonably well with a cane and fifty degrees of bend as well as lifting three pounds of weight on my ankle. Success is not being dead or more seriously crippled.

◆   ◆   ◆

Or losing my leg.

I began the process of lowering my benchmarks or changing them, as Michael said. I think it will be a long time before I'm ready to see this as just a change and not a handicap or disability. All too clearly, I still see the things I can't do because of the inhibited function of my leg, and there are no real benefits to this. There are no sudden new skills I can master because of the change in my body.

There is nothing beyond the simple fact that I didn't die. Whatever changes this has wrought in me, they were necessary, or my life would likely have ended. I guess that's a pretty potent benefit right there.

Fiveteen
Winter and Work

So, I continued the long, agonizing process of retraining my damaged flesh to accept its new self in order to adapt and bend. Breaking down the scar tissue and the adhesions, learning how to walk again, and getting to that magical fifty degrees of bend took four months of two-hour workouts per day, five days a week. When we reached it, the focus changed. We were no longer trying to push the limits of what I could do; we were merely trying to maintain it. Joanne changed my schedule to three days a week and then two.

One day, she was talking to a student about me and commented about my cancer as having been aggressive. It brought me up short. Really? It wasn't something I had realized. It was also a thought I had not allowed. She said, "Look what they did to you to fight it." When I mentioned this to people, they said they suspected as much. My speedy passage through the medical system boded seriously for my condition. I suppose I must have known it, but I don't honestly think I could have dealt with that. Everyone I dealt with was calm; therefore everything was going to be all right. The mind's ability to reduce things and make them manageable is amazing.

I continued seeing Jon Hunter every month. If it was difficult to talk to people who didn't understand the language of the disease, it was always easy to talk to Jon. He speaks fluent cancer. It's what his practice is based on. When I was hard on myself, he made me see it and helped me ease it. When I was angry, I could be angry, and he always understood why. He was never shy about telling me when I was shortchanging my own trauma and pain, and he could always focus on what I was saying and get at the nugget of truth buried in it. On my first visit, when he offered his hand to shake at the end of the session, on an impulse, I hugged him because my intuition told me it was right. Every session since has ended the same way.

On one of these visits, we discussed how I sometimes felt the leg was not a part of me. I looked at it, wiggled my toes, and knew intellectually it was still my leg. But I didn't feel like it was real or a part of me. He described it as a variant of phantom limb syndrome. My mental picture of the leg I had before was so strong and so deeply ingrained that it would take a long time to become accustomed to how it is now.

I visited Peter Satok often as well, touching base and keeping him informed of the progress or the stasis, depending on how I was feeling at the time. He once said, "You've done well." It was like receiving the Nobel Peace prize.

As autumn waned and crept toward winter, my disability, sick leave, vacation days, and all various sources of income began drying up. I began thinking about returning to work. It was something I needed for my sanity as much as my bank account. I had spent so much time on my back while I healed and so much time away from the world and people that I craved the stimulation again.

The question was, "Where and how?" My store was gone. Gutted and reno-vated, it bore no relation to the store I had helped run. Margot had left. The staff had so disliked her replacement that they were almost all gone as well. The loss of the store cut deeply. It had given me a place to work when I arrived. It had taken me in and provided opportunities for advancement. When Kerry and I split up, it gave me an anchor that helped me hold on to Toronto and not give up and leave. When I got sick, it gave me someplace to look forward to returning. Now, I was ready to return to work, and there was nowhere to return.

As luck would have it, I was in the Eaton Centre one day, having just come from physiotherapy. I was in the Smithbooks #327 on the third level that had been our good-natured rival during my time at Store #3. I had stopped to say hello to the few friends I had that worked there. While there, the phone rang for the manager, Brad. I heard him mention my name, telling whoever was on the line that I was in the store. It was our regional manager, and I was summoned to the phone to discuss my plans for returning to work.

I was assigned to Brad and #327. It would be part-time in what amounted to a seasonal position for the upcoming Christmas season. In the few days before I actu-ally walked through the door for the first time, I felt a new fear at the prospect of returning and the challenges that might arise. What if I failed? What if I couldn't do it? What then? But the feelings had to be faced. I had to try. On that first day, I discovered my new role. When I had left, I was the assistant manager. Now, I was to man the cash desk. I was given a stool to sit on. I was basically treated like I was made of blown glass and would shatter if stressed in the slightest.

Though it rankled (think of my tendency to hate being coddled), it was kind and considerate of them, considering the ordeal I had just been through. In many ways, I was still in a few shades of denial about just how horrific it had all been. The constant hesitation to not push me in any way was irritating.

So, I settled in behind the cash desk, rang in purchases, and sold loyalty cards. The shifts were short at the start, which was good because I tired easily. It had been a long time since I had put in that kind of time at work. My leg ached, resonating all along the bonds between bone and metal. The intense physical and emotional trauma had left me weaker than I suspected, but my stamina slowly increased. It felt good to be back in an arena I cared about.

Business intensified as winter came, gearing up toward the insanity that is an Eaton Centre Christmas. The snow came, slushy and thick, bringing a whole new set of adaptation issues. Ridges of ploughed, dirty snow appeared at the curbs of intersections, making them grimy and treacherous. (Snow is pristine and white in Toronto for about a half hour before it begins turning brown). I learned how to negotiate these mounds with my leg that only bent at fifty degrees. Ice and slippery snow became less of a concern than I thought they would be. My new gait, slower and more deliberate, minimized the chances of a slip and fall.

The crowds in the mall continued increasing as Christmas neared. It didn't bother me much because I had already experienced two Eaton Centre Christmases and had a reasonably good handle on coping. You just need to relax and do what you can. The calmer you stay, the calmer the crowd stays. I'm also that rare genetic throwback who actually enjoys the customer service environment. I like helping people find what they need and leave my place of business with a smile on their faces.

Sadly, as Christmas neared, _____ and I came to a quiet end. As I became somewhat more sure of myself and as my body and mind continued healing, I realized no one in his life knew I existed. No one in his family or any of his friends were aware of me. In fact, one of his closest friends visited, and he didn't even make the slightest effort to introduce us. He just said he could see me again when she was gone. When that happened, something died in my heart. I knew I couldn't continue with the relationship. He said he didn't think he could be my friend, so I don't see him anymore except when I accidentally run into him. I've thought a lot about it in the time that has passed, especially in the light of later events. I don't know if I just fell in love with him because I needed to be in love to ease the pain and needed to feel that someone could love me. But he was there for me during a horrible time. Even if it was doomed from the start, it made my recuperation easier. I'll always be grateful to him for that.

One day, as I was talking to a coworker, a new reaction appeared, a new voice in response to my illness. Poor Jeff had been dumped by a girl he truly cared for and was hurt and confused. At various times, I think he talked to all of us about what he was feeling. But, when he talked to me, I was the perfect listener on the surface, attentive and compassionate. Inside, I only wanted to smash his head against the wall and scream until he understood what had happened to me, showing him the great cosmic scale of suffering and how being dumped came nowhere close to what I had been through. In the end, composure won out. That particular madness seethed unheard.

The season sped by. By the time I found out I had four days off over Christmas, it was too late and too expensive to fly home. My Christmas celebration that year was a quiet dinner with Gordon, David, and David's sister, Alison, which was fine and apropos. Gordon is as close to me as the brother I never had. We talked and laughed. There was wine and good food. All of the essential elements were there.

When I returned to work after my holiday break, new hints and rumblings were in the air. The gods of book retail, denied the slaughter of Store #3, demanded a sacrifice once again. This time, they would not be denied. At the end of January, Store #327 would close forever. Unlike the previous spring, there would be no eleventh-hour reprieve. The official announcement was made. The main sales area was roped off, and the process of returns began. Any books too worn to be returned were marked down 50 percent. My job expanded to include the branding of these books with red stickers for the sale tables at the front of the store.

While we presided over the sad dismantling of the store, the battle for control of Chapters began. Heather Reisman of Indigo made her play for control of the company. Larry Stevenson countered with the support of Future Shop. When the dust settled, Indigo controlled. We were absorbed into a new corporate umbrella as the merger progressed, but we were too busy emptying shelves and dismantling fixtures to really take note. There's something incredibly forlorn about picking apart the corpse of a store like that and watching it get emptier and shabbier.

I was one of the lucky ones as the end drew near. I received an offer to transfer to Store #585 on Queen Street East in the Beach neighbourhood. I had a place to go. On top of that, I liked the area and the store. In fact, I had semijoked with the regional manager about wanting to take it over. I don't know if that was her intention, as circumstances steered us all away from that, but I was comfortable with where I was headed next.

As I was ticketing the damaged books, I had the perfect opportunity to skim a few off the top for myself. They were being discounted anyway. What was the difference if or someone else bought them? The most frequently damaged types of book are the computer titles. They are the most needed and among the most expensive. Rather than buy them, people browse them for the piece of information they need and put them back. I stashed a couple of HTML books aside as the idea occurred to me to create a Web site. I had space included in my high-speed Internet package, and it seemed like the time to put it to use. I knew the books would help me with the coding, even though I did most of the original work with Netscape Composer by just opening the program and playing. While we were destroying the store, I was planning, designing, and writing content for my site. Eventually, I uploaded it. It's still running today, if modified more than once. My Web presence was born.

Then, one day at the end of January, the last returnable books had been returned, and the remaining sale stock was reduced by 75 percent and blown out the door. I showed up for what was supposed to be my last shift and discovered there was nothing for me to do. I was sent to another store in the PATH under downtown Toronto, where the manager needed extra help that day. And Smith-books #327, Level 3 of the Eaton Centre, was gone.

◆   ◆   ◆

The Beaches (or The Beach, depending on who you talk to) is like a small town hidden in a big city. It rides the border between Metro Toronto and Scar-borough along the edge of Lake Ontario. The people who live there are a curious mix of those who have lived there for years and the nouveau riche who are among the few who can afford to live there. Any given afternoon will find the streets full of women who can afford not to work, pushing baby carriages that cost as much as compact cars. Dogs are everywhere. Any savvy business owner who can legally get away with it allows dogs in the store and keeps dog biscuits behind the counter.

Tucked among the tourist stores and fancy decorating places, next to the liquor store and across the street from the Shopper's Drug Mart, is Smithbooks #585. I think it's the only store of that format that isn't in a mall.

This was to be the new base of operations where I would hang my hat. I worked with Jen, the manager who had been with the company for years and who trekked in from Etobicoke everyday. I worked with Aylsa, who had lived just up the street her whole life and still lived in the house where she grew up. Sandra, who dressed in black from head to toe, wore cocksucker red lipstick, loathed garlic, and had a per-verse fascination with blood. (If I hadn't seen her reflection in a mirror, I would have been frightened.) Lindsay, who was nineteen going on forty, loved white zin-fandel and pierogies at parties. I swear she talked faster than anyone I knew. I immediately felt at home. Jen was glad to have me because I came already trained and had strong book knowledge and customer service skills. Within a week or so, I had made Sandra blush, something she usually did to others.

The regular customers took me to their hearts as well. For them, that location wasn't an outlet or a corporate representative. This was their neighbourhood bookstore where they bought their *New York Times* on Sunday and dropped in to browse on their evening walk with the dog. To be a part of that store, you had to become a part of the community, and I needed to be a part of a community that had nothing to do with hospitals or treatment. A community of everyday, non-cancer people was exactly what I needed.

Unfortunately, there was never any real escape. Not even a month after my move, I received word from Carole that Julie had died. She had not reached her twentieth birthday, and her fight was over.

Strangely, I didn't grieve much when I heard. I think I grieved in the fall when I learned it was coming and my survivor's guilt had torn me open. Now, I only felt relief she was at peace. There would be no more punishing treatments or pain for her. If she couldn't have health, she could at least have rest. I wrote this for my Web site, after recounting how Carole and Julie had come into my life, how I had heard Julie's lovely voice singing in the patient lounge at the hospital:

> *"Today my heart is big and sore*
> *it's trying to push right through my skin."*
> *~Patty Griffin~*
> *"Good-bye"*

The last time I saw Carole was in the fall when I was on the verge of giving up my crutches and switching to my cane. I was visiting another patient in my old room, at the behest of one of my nurses, a young man whose lower leg had been amputated. I walked around the corner, and she was with her husband. She came rushing up and gave me a great big hug. She was cryptic that day, saying they and the doctors were discussing decisions that had to be made about Julie.

On September 19, Linda forwarded me an e-mail from Carole. Julie's cancer was inoperable. They could only make her comfortable and let her go. My own traumas still so fresh, I wept for what seemed like a couple of solid days. How could I ever face Carole again, knowing the disease I had beaten was going to kill her daughter? I felt burning, deep shame that I was going to live and this beautiful child was not. If there had been some way, at that moment, I would have happily given Julie my remaining years. But those sentiments are spurious and hollow. There is no machine to transfer life force. There is no magic spell. The dice had been rolled.

Carole kept in touch. They went on a cruise and took Julie to Disney World. They made every second count, as far as I could tell, as far as that is possible.

On February 23, after five-and-a-half weeks in the hospital, Julie died. (You must forgive my bluntness. I've never liked euphemisms like "passed away" or "left us.") I shed a few tears, but I don't think it's really hit me yet. My own ups and downs over the last few years have left me exhausted. My feelings now are for Carole and the rest of her family. Julie's suffering is now over, but their grief will last a long while. I wish there was something I could do to ease her pain and soothe the coming days. But she is miles away, and I don't think she's ready for contact with me. Deep inside, I still feel the terrible weight of this survivor's guilt that I have survived. Like grief, I guess this too shall pass. Sleep well, Julie. You faced the horrors with a courage beyond your years.

> *"And I wonder where you are*
> *and if the pain ends, when you die.*
> *And I wonder if there was*
> *some better way to say*
> *goodbye."*
> *~Patty Griffin~*
> *"Good-bye"*

I sent an e-mail to Carole to let her know I was thinking of her and she could contact me whenever she felt ready. She eventually told me she printed off what I had written and placed it with her collection of memories of Julie. She said I should never feel guilty or think she would blame me for surviving when Julie had not. She told me she was deeply happy I was well.

◆   ◆   ◆

As they inevitably do, the seasons changed again. Spring came. Though I felt happy and safe at the store, I thought a better-paying job might be out there. My time on disability had left me with a large debt. Though I loved books and the store, I reluctantly thought it might be time for a change. I spoke with an employment counselor Kerry put me in contact with. She connected me with a job interview for a call centre at one of the major banks, handling credit card inquiries. After one of those spectacularly irritating, behaviour-based interviews ("Tell me about a situation in which you…"), I received a phone call informing me the interview had revealed I couldn't handle the stress (?!?!?!?!?). I tabled thoughts of a major career change and concentrated on my life as it was.

After my tax refund arrived that spring, I could travel home for the first time since becoming ill. The first time through security was interesting when my knee set off the metal detectors. It was also interesting sitting in the cramped seat with a leg that wouldn't bend properly. But I made it. I landed in Regina on April 1. When I stepped out of the airport, the quiet stopped me dead. It stunned me because I had grown so accustomed to the general background noise of Toronto.

On that trip, I turned thirty-eight. I saw my family, and I was pampered. In their eyes and manner, I could see they were haunted as well. My struggle back to life had taken a toll on them. I reconnected with my friends and told the story over coffee and lunch many times, rolling up the legs of my pants to show the scar. Eventually, I grew tired of hearing the words coming from my mouth.

I think there's something necessary to actually spending time with loved ones after something like this happens. When you're recovered, they need to see you and touch you. If you shimmered out of existence for a while, they need to be reminded you're real and okay. It's something you need as well, especially if your illness occurred out of their field of vision. That spring, we all reassured each other that I had indeed survived and still existed.

When I returned, I wrote this on my Web site:

◆   ◆   ◆

Home, there's an emotionally loaded word for you. It's funny, When I told people here I was going to be away, I told them I was going home. Then, as my holiday was winding down, I told people there that I was ready to go home (meaning here in Toronto). A friend of mine asked, "Is home just the place you aren't?"

My trip began with a flight into Regina. My sister Jennifer picked me up and drove me to the parental house in Moose Jaw. The house hasn't changed much, having completed most of its metamorphoses since I moved away to school in 1981. I know it's the house I grew up in, but my parents have changed it so much that it's become their house, not our house.

I relaxed for the first few days—sleeping late, reading, doing crossword puzzles, and just reveling in the fact that, for the first time in two years, there was nowhere I had to be. There were no doctors to see, no physiotherapy, and no radiation. I had nothing to do with my illness or recovery. I spent time with the few people I'm still in contact with from my high school days. I spent just enough time there to realize just how hellish it would be to be a gay man living in Moose Jaw, buried so deeply in the closet that you might never see daylight, or to declare yourself and maybe never feel accepted at home. I was ready to go to Saskatoon when my birthday rolled around, or so I thought. My parents drove me up on the Friday, and we had dinner with my sister Linda. After dropping my things off at my friend Kim's place, where I was staying, I jaunted down to Diva's, the one gay bar in town. I wanted to see the owner, who I had known for years, and anyone else who crossed my path. I had barely sat down on the upper balcony when my friend Mike came in. He took one look at me, broke into a huge smile, and bounded up the stairs and into my arms. I've noticed that's the way with old friends, those people whose souls are welded deep inside of us. You can spend years apart, and, the instant you see each other again, it's like no time has passed.

It was like that with each person I spent time—Kim, Suzanne, Scott, Gillian, Dan, Penny, and Sandra. It was as if it had been merely days, instead of years, had passed between us. Even the people I ran into by accident, the ones I had lost track of, they were miraculously there as I went to and from engagements. It's a lovely experience to be face-to-face with people who genuinely love you and are glad to see you.

I soon discovered, when one has survived a life-threatening experience, there is this intense edge to peoples' happiness when they see you for the first time. If you couple that with having to dredge up the details and repeatedly show off the scar, you will see how I was drained by the end of the two weeks.

More than that, I found myself feeling self-conscious in front of all of these people who only knew the old, unhandicapped me. They were seeing the new postcancer me for the first time. It was easy to start thinking, feeling, and reacting like the old me, the one who used sex and sexual attraction for validation, the one who often sat alone at the bar and just watched, and the insecure one who was always sure no one would ever find him attractive.

At the end of the two weeks, I was ready to come back to Toronto and be me—the me I have become—again. Even though I had only been home for a few days, I felt more like the me I have become since my illness. This is the battleground where I built a life after Kerry and I split, where I fought cancer and won. For now, I don't belong in Saskatchewan, even though my family and several dear friends are there. I said to my friend Beth that I've always been a person for whom home was about a molecule or two bigger than my skin. I've always worked to create home wherever I was. Maybe I just had to leave home to find home.

◆   ◆   ◆

The first time I saw Joanne after I returned to Toronto, I discovered I had somehow gained another three degrees of bend. When she measured, I was at fifty-three degrees. I went a few more times, and the extra flexibility remained. Nine months after the process had started, she discharged me. Despite there were still regular checkups, X-rays, and continual monitoring, I felt I had crossed the Rubicon. I began to feel, if not whole (I would never feel that again), at least like the worst of the storm had passed.

Dr. Wunder had mentioned the odds of nonlocal recurrence for synovial sarcomas were 30–70 percent. I knew it might happen, but I was getting better everyday. I was happy at the store. My life began feeling like my own again.

Around that time, as May was blooming, my favourite singer in the world, Eddi Reader, appeared at the Horseshoe Tavern on Queen Street West. It was her only Canadian stop on the tour. She was opening for some other band I didn't care about. She played an hour-long acoustic set, and I had to stand because no seats were left. But I didn't care. If I had to, I would have hung from the rafters. She sang every bit as beautifully in person as she did on CD. She stayed after her set and spoke to anyone who wanted to meet her and get signed CDs. I told her how much her music meant to me and it had gotten me through my cancer. I told her I had been cancer-free for a year. She beamed and flung her arms around me. I think I floated home that night.

The anniversary of my surgery was approaching, and I knew I should do something to celebrate my health and life. I thought about holding a cocktail party. As it turned out, I had to work. I needed the money too much to get rid of my shift. In the end, the day was just ordinary. I got up and read the paper with my cup of coffee. I went to work, and nothing eventful happened. After work, on my way home, I realized it was exactly what I needed. After the past year, I just needed nothing dramatic to happen.

Still, I wanted to do something that would mark the achievement. The idea of getting a tattoo had always intrigued me. I had just never known what to get. The foremost possibility was the Red Dragon symbol in mah jongg. I've always loved the shape of the symbol, even though I hesitated because I didn't really know what it meant. But I kept coming back to it. So, after some Internet searching, I discovered one of the meanings was "to hit a target" or "to attain." It was settled. I had it tattooed on my chest in black and highlighted in red. People asked if it hurt. I told them, comparatively, no!

I had come full circle. I had recovered from a horrible experience and rebuilt my life. What I didn't know was that another meaning of the symbol was "middle."

Sixteen
Chemotherapy

On a recent trip home, I wrote this next part of the story. Writing of my diagnosis and the subsequent events flowed from me after the initial surgery, but the flow stopped. I felt the story was over. I was too preoccupied with my life as it had become. It was the life of, as Jon Hunter stated, "I'm not going to die, now what?" When my cancer recurred, I had no strength or will to write. Only recently, the fire burned again, and I felt the need to finish telling the story. On this particular trip, I found a café. One afternoon, I picked up my fountain pen and a ratty notebook. The words flowed anew.

On the second day, when I knew I was going to write about this next stage in the war, I became physically ill. When my mind realized the Pandora's box it was going to open, it sent the message through my body. While at lunch with my dear friend Penny, my stomach began bothering me as we were finishing up the meal. I excused myself to go to the washroom and promptly vomited through my mouth and nose. That simple, natural act suddenly brought back the emotional trauma of my first recurrence. I took two Gravol, went back to the café where I found my muse again, and picked up my pen. If this book was a map, this chapter would be dark and shadowed with a label reading, "Here be dragons."

That spring and summer brought more changes. Dave decided to move out. I don't remember why. I saw him once after that when he picked up something he left behind. I guess our season ended. As it turned out, Gordon and David needed a place because the house they were renting was going to be sold. David was leaving for school in Iowa that fall, so they moved in, intending for Gordon to stay behind in Toronto while he was gone. A few months later, Pauline left as well, and Eleanor took her place. I've lived that way for years as roommates replaced roommates. There was little trauma involved.

I had terminated my sessions with Jon Hunter. In typical laid-back Jon fashion, he looked at me one day and said something like, "What are you still doing here? You don't need me anymore!" It was true. I felt like I had turned the corner and was on the way to being healthy and strong again. He had helped me face my feelings and realize I had come through it.

That May, I went for another X-ray and another follow-up appointment at Dr. Wunder's sarcoma clinic. In the year since the surgery on my leg, I had grown accustomed to these tests. Three months before, there had been an X-ray. It was normal. Every X-ray until then had been normal. It was all standard operating procedure.

When the door opened on the beige room that day, the resident du jour was there. Doctors have a studied, careful way of speaking and a skill for giving you information in small, neutral doses that are never false. However, they are ever so careful of your feelings so they don't always hit the truth.

The X-ray showed something. That bit of doctor-speak was my first clue. He spoke of scar tissue or possibly a shadow on the film. As before, I accepted the announcement at face value. He didn't seem alarmed. Why should I be? He didn't mention recurrence at that point, and hope can be a persistent thing. A CT, always more detailed, was arranged for June 27. Another appointment was set for July 3.

The possibility of recurrence entered my mind. I told my friends, family, and coworkers, stressing the shred of hope that was the only thing keeping me going. We didn't know, and there was no point falling to pieces until we did know. I grasped at that straw and held it tight until it begged for mercy. We didn't know.

Somewhere deep inside, I did know (or at least suspected) what the news would be when I returned. I was all too aware of that 30–70 percent chance of lung recurrence. They weren't the best of odds, and the deck was definitely stacked against me. I was hopeful but cautious. Once the unthinkable happens to you once, it isn't so unthinkable anymore. I knew, if I went into that next appointment and received the news I was semiexpecting, I wanted someone there with me. I asked Gordon to come.

On the morning of July 3, I dutifully reported to the sarcoma clinic on the fourth floor of Princess Margaret Hospital. As we waited, I filled out my questionnaire on my abilities and responses to my illness. (One of the people on Jay Wunder's team is Anthony Griffin. He compiles research on how people cope with their illness and how they describe the changes brought on by it. My running joke with him is that I mark responses at random just to skew the curve.) I was ushered into the beige, blank cubicle to wait.

As before, Dr. Wunder broke the news. The CT had confirmed the presence of several cancerous nodules in my lungs. The final count was eight: three on the right side and five on the left. They were all small. The largest was about a centimetre. All were all in operable locations. (Medicine's knowledge of the lungs and how they work is extensive. They know which bits they can take out and how the various areas are supplied with blood. The road map is a detailed one.)

Dr. Wunder was kind and gentle in delivering this blow. He apologetically asked if he could bring in his new resident or visiting surgeon. (I can't remember which.) I guess I was still, even in my newly diseased state, a textbook case of a Kotz prosthesis surgery waiting to be studied. In my stunned state, I said yes. What I had been through was something this new doctor might never see again. I don't think I ever lost sight of that, regardless of what was happening.

As luck would have it, the oncologist who took over my care could see me in his own clinic that very day. I was ushered through a couple of halls into another beige examination room. The first thing I did was hand Gordon my cancer journal and a pen to take notes. Despite my outer calm, I knew I was in shock and would probably not remember much of what was I was told that day. The one thing I remember is how easy it was to slip back into the mind-set of being ready to fight, that is, slip on the gloves and put up my dukes.

A doctor working with the oncologist gave me my introductory course in Chemotherapy 101. The only thing I remember about her was her Australian accent.

The premise behind chemotherapy is brutally simple. No agent can specifically kill cancer cells. What can be targeted are fast-growing cells, which cancer cells are. The patient is treated with one or a combination of highly toxic chemicals to try to shrink tumours by killing the fast-growing cancer cells. Unfortunately, this attack is indiscriminate. Fast-growing cells also affected include the cells of your hair follicles. This is why your hair falls out. It's not just the hair on your head. It's from all over your body. It's all gone. The cells lining your gastrointestinal tract and mucous membranes are destroyed as well. (Mouth sores are a potential side effect.) Also, your white blood cells, which inhibit your body's ability to fight infections, are gone. Even your sperm production cells are destroyed, rendering you infertile. The nice woman told me I should bank sperm if I ever planned to have children. When I said it wasn't likely, she just smiled gently and said, "I kind of got that idea, but I had to ask."

With the basic course under my belt, I met Dr. Martin Blackstein, the man who would oversee my poisoning. Other patients I've talked to who would tell you he does not have any bedside manner. I would be hard pressed to disagree. Dr. Blackstein is fairly no-nonsense, and there is nothing touchy-feely to him. Only disease, treatment, and results are in his world. However, he knows what he is doing, and that is the bottom line. (As before, Dr. Satok had worked with Dr. Blackstein at one point and said he trusted him. That was good enough for me.)

Dr. Blackstein provided more information. He said, if the CT showed us eight nodules, there were undoubtedly more. They were too small to be visible. The purpose of the chemo was to attack these as well as shrink the visible ones. The regimen I would be given was a combination of Doxorubicin (Gordon would write Doxarheumacyn in his notes) and Ifosfamide. It was a particularly aggressive combination. The chemo would be inpatient. (I would be admitted to the hospital for two to three days while the drugs were administered). Depending on my response to the drugs, there would be five or six cycles. Each cycle would be three weeks apart. Between each cycle, I would rest and regain my strength. There would be blood work each week and a weeklong cycle of Ciprofloxacin, an antibiotic to prevent any infections my weakened immune system couldn't handle. If I developed a fever at any time, I was to report to emergency immediately. There could be no alcohol or sunlight. The drugs could accumulate in my skin and stain if exposed to the sun. It was highly unlikely I would be able to work.

When my scant questions were answered, I was sent on my way. When they knew the start date of the first cycle, they would call me. In the meantime, there were more tests. On July 5, I went to nuclear medicine at Mount Sinai for something called a MUGA scan. I was injected with a radioactive substance to test my heart. The Doxorubicin had the potential to damage my heart if the dose and duration were high enough. Dr. Blackstein wasn't worried about it at the level I would receive, but it was a necessary precaution. After that, on July 8, I had a bone scan to ensure there was no presence of cancer there. I lay on the machine's platform for more than a half hour as the scanner skimmed over my entire body, barely an inch or two from my skin.

A familiar pattern occurred in the days following the news of this recurrence. I informed everyone and made what plans I could. As I mentioned, it was surprisingly easy to slip back into fighting mode, but I also did what I had done before. I made it smaller, that is, I made it seem like it was easier than it was. I could cope if it was smaller, less dramatic, and less intrusive. The tumours were small. They were operable. It was fine.

One of the first things I did was phone Mike Forbes in Winnipeg and tell him. Of anyone in my life, Mike would understand. He had undergone a course of chemo after the amputation of his foot. Each cycle was a different drug or combination of drugs. He eventually said the Doxo/Ifos had been the worst. We talked on the phone often, like twins who shared a language that no one else understood.

When I told the girls at work, Jen made sure I knew my place at the store was secure. When I was better, I could return. I needed to know that. After the loss of my old store the last time, I needed to feel there was a safe place to return.

All too soon, I received the call. My first cycle of chemo would begin on July 11. Despite my resolve to fight and my deployment of every coping skill I had, the terror surged that day when I arrived at the temporary location of the oncology clinic. Despite the fact I had fought the disease once and had beaten it back, that experience was, in many ways, irrelevant. This was all new. There was nothing familiar. It was a cruel irony. I was fighting the same disease in a completely different way. All was horrible and new with no signposts or landmarks. The waiting area was filled with people in various stages of treatment. Some looked reasonably well. Others were desperately ill. My stomach churned.

Blood was taken. An IV saline lock was put in. I was sent to X-ray. When I returned, Dr. Blackstein saw me, and we talked about what was coming. Then I went to the main floor to be admitted. I returned to the eleventh floor, the same floor I had been just over a year before. The first nurse I saw was Pat, who had cared for me while training Jane. The other nurse was Suzette, who had a sweet smile and the traces of an exotic accent.

That first time, I was given a semiprivate room that my insurance from work paid for. They hooked me up to the IV and began the pretreatment. There were the antinauseants, Granesitron and a steroid called Dexamethisone. Something called Mesna protected my bladder from the toxicity of the Doxorubicin. It was combined with lots of fluid to keep my bladder clear. With these in my system, it was time for my poisoning.

Doxorubicin is a vile drug. It is bloody, Kool-Aid red in colour. It is administered in a slow twenty-minute push into the IV line. If it went any faster, it would eat away at the inside of my vein. That first day, Suzette sat and talked with me. On other days, depending on my mood, there was either talk or silence with other nurses.

After the Doxo, I had more fluids and diuretics to keep my system from flushing the chemo drugs. I spent a large amount of that first day up and down to the bathroom, which was difficult because my mobility was still limited, especially with the extra burden of the IV pole to move with me.

The Ifosfamide in a slow, twenty-four hour drip was next. I would read, rest, pee, or talk to whoever was visiting. Mostly, I just waited and experienced one of the more odd side effects that would plague me for the full chemo course. For some reason, around 50 percent of chemo patients get hiccups. My bouts were violent and lasted around twenty to forty minutes each and every cycle.

After the Ifos, there were more antinauseants, more Mesna, and more fluids. On Friday morning, it was all disconnected. I was free to go home. I was given a prescription for the Cipro and two requisitions for blood work to be done on the subsequent Wednesdays. The results were to be faxed to Dr. Blackstein's office. After a short, half hour session with Jon Hunter, I caught a cab home and collapsed on the couch.

That first cycle, I felt lousy. It was like I had a horrible flu that laid me up, weak and exhausted. It was like a truck had run over me. But there was no vomiting. I wasn't altogether surprised at that. Dr. Blackstein assured me I was getting the "gold standard" of antinausea drugs. Plus, I tend to have a cast iron stomach. It takes nothing short of food poisoning to make me throw up. For whatever reason, I was glad to have been spared. The chemo was decidedly unpleasant, but, if that was what I could expect, I could tolerate four or five more of these treatments. Little did I know.

I didn't move much the rest of that Friday or, for that matter, over that first weekend. As the weekend progressed, that sick, hungover, flu-like feeling began fading. On Tuesday, July 17, I travelled to Princess Margaret once again and met Dr. Michael Johnston, the thoracic surgeon who would remove the nodules from my lungs, for the first time.

Jon Hunter referred to Dr. Johnston as "a bit of an ice man, but a damn good surgeon." That worked for me. I didn't need another friend. I needed a surgeon who could open me up and excise the cancer from my body. When I met him, he didn't seem at all like an ice man. He was just good-natured and like a dad in that slightly detached, 1950s-sitcom dad kind of way. He outlined the procedure he would perform. He would open my chest and saw through my sternum, opening my chest cavity. First on one lung and then the other, he would remove the tumours, taking conical sections of tissue around them and closing the lung around the space. Once I was released from the hospital, there was one strict rule of no pushing, pulling, or lifting for four to six weeks. When he was finished and had left the room, his associate, Dr. Jugnauth, answered my one frivolous concern. My tattoo would be undamaged!

By Wednesday, I felt almost normal. I was slower and more tired. It was like I had a full body bruise. The body remembers, and the footprint of those drugs went deep. I left the house and found a lab to take my blood.

My days after the chemo were similar to the days of recovery from the leg surgery. Daytime TV…Donny and Marie…Stand-up comedians. After lunch, I went to the Tango Palace and curled up with a book for hours. The guys there all knew what was happening and let me stay as long as I wanted. The evenings were quiet. I usually spent time on my computer or watching TV. As my strength came back, I visited the store.

Just as I felt something like my old self again, it was time for the next cycle. Another of those massive ironies of cancer is that I felt fine when they told me of the mets in my lungs. There was no pain, shortness of breath, or sensations at all. It was only when they began treatment that I began to wish I was dead.

Once again, I went on disability, but I took another blow when I discovered my new claim was an even smaller portion of my salary because I had been working reduced hours in the intervening year. At nearly forty years of age, I lived for months on money my family sent.

I reported back for my second chemo cycle on August 1. It was the same procedure. This time, there wasn't a semiprivate room, so I stayed in the mini chemo ward. It was four rooms with sliding walls that partitioned the beds. It was more like having a room to myself. That first day, the faces of the nurses and the patients in the other beds was the only thing different.

On Thursday morning, deep in the Ifos, the significant change became apparent. I was beginning to feel the full force of the nausea when I woke. When breakfast came, I wasn't feeling very hungry. The only thing that appealed to me was strawberry yogurt, so that was all I ate. Within fifteen minutes, I had my first chemo vomit…in pretty, Barbie doll pink. My cast iron innards had failed me.

The nurse that morning, Jose, emptied the basin and offered me a Popsicle. They apparently help with the nausea and are easy on the ravaged digestive tract. Within minutes, I had my second chemo vomit in grape-synthetic purple. Fearing food for the first time in my life, I asked for ginger ale. My third chemo vomit was amber gold. Even water came back up. I gave up trying to ingest anything.

During that awful Thursday, Kim visited. She was in town with friends on the one weekend I wasn't free. She brought a book, *Bellwether*, by Connie Willis. I thanked her, and we talked a few minutes, arranging a visit on the weekend once I was home. I said good-bye by waving her toward the door as a spasm of vomiting overcame me. I couldn't stand the thought of her seeing me like that. Thankfully, the pattern of vomiting was established that day when it ceased after about a half hour.

The nausea that followed me home that Friday was worse and grew cumulatively as the level of poison in my system increased and the damage worsened. But I had another three-week reprieve.

During that break, I reached up to run my hand over my goatee (a tic I developed a long time ago), and a scrap of hair came away, leaving a naked patch of bare skin. Within the next few weeks, eyebrows, eyelashes, nose hair, and pubic hair disappeared. Only a smattering of the hair on my chest remained. Perversely, the hair on my back, the one place I would happily have lost it, remained!

Several smart-asses thought it was funny to comment, because I shaved my head, I "had no hair to lose." I never found it funny. Believe me, you will miss your eyelashes when they're gone. Every bit of dust or airborne thing will get in your eyes. Without your nose hair, those same contaminants will have your nose constantly running.

My GI tract suffered as well. I became constipated from the drugs, and the damage to my mucous membranes left me with bleeding haemorrhoids. Every bowel movement was like passing shards of broken glass. The toilet tissue came away bloody red, as if the Doxorubicin had somehow torn its way through my body and was exiting unmetabolized.

The lingering nausea grew steadily worse. Though I only vomited during that Thursday morning of the actual cycle, the dragging, debilitating, "sick" feeling stayed. Imagine the worst flu you've ever had or the worst hangover. Multiply it by twenty. Imagine it in every cell, muscle, and bone. It's pervasive and punishing. It only really leaves you in the last week before you have to go back. Then you begin dreading what you know is coming.

The fact I was helpless worsened it. There was nothing I could do except show up. When I was recovering from the surgery on my leg, my recovery at least depended somewhat on my effort and input. Now there was nothing I could do except hang on with my fingernails while they tore in the dirt of the cliff face.

Before my third cycle began on August 22, I was back in radiology, having another PIC line inserted. In the first and second cycles, whenever I moved the arm with the saline lock into certain positions, the IV would occlude, setting off an alarm on the metre measuring the dose into my system. (To this day, the sound of one of those alarms makes the hairs on the back of my neck stand up if I hear it in the hospital.) The nurses asked Dr. Blackstein if the PIC line could be inserted to avoid this and make the process easier and avoid any potential venous damage from the Doxorubicin. I hated the idea. It meant another home care nurse checking the dressing and flushing it daily. It made me feel as if I was going backward, not forward. In the end, I lost the fight. Though I wasn't happy about it, I knew it was a good idea. Once more, the flexible silicone tube was inserted in my arm, trailing deep into me before ending up near my heart. I still have the two tiny scars on my bicep from those procedures.

During that third cycle, I thought I would outwit the nausea. I didn't eat anything after my breakfast on the Wednesday. It didn't make a difference. Despite there being no food in my stomach (thus no pretty colours), the poison would not be denied. Right on schedule, Thursday morning and for nearly the same length of time, I vomited clear bile several times.

During that third cycle, I noticed something that gave me hope and kept me going. The cancer gods had granted me a boon. My injured leg was bending better. In fact, it was noticeably and dramatically better. Joanne visited and noticed, telling me to come by the physiotherapy gym for an official measurement when I felt up to it. It showed more than seventy degrees. We've never figured out why. We tossed around the theory that the chemotherapy somehow loosened the adhesions between the scar tissue and the healthy tissue. It might have been just sheer bullheaded stubbornness. It might have been the same good genes that were causing the chemo to have a dramatic, rapid effect in visibly shrinking the tumours on the X-rays. I don't think we'll ever know. The horrible side effects were worth it because the drugs were doing their job.

When I had been diagnosed with the mets in my lungs, I began sessions again with Jon Hunter. After a brief meeting the morning after my first chemo, we had our next session the day before my fourth cycle of chemo was to begin.

On September 11, 2001…

Seventeen
9/11

Like the generation before mine, who can tell you exactly where they were when they heard of John Kennedy's assassination, our generation will be able to say just where they were when they heard the World Trade Center had fallen.

I was at Mount Sinai Hospital. I had just come from an appointment with Jon Hunter, our first full session after my recurrence and descent into chemotherapy. We talked about how I felt emotionally and physically. It was a feeling of utter betrayal. I had done everything right. I fought hard and was strong. I opened up to friends and accepted their help. I didn't give in to the despair. Yet, here I was again. The disease was eating at me, and I was enduring brutal chemotherapy to try to keep me alive. But at the same time there was the sense that there was nothing to feel betrayed by. There was no source or cause of this imagined treachery. How do you feel betrayed by a disease? It knows nothing of how you struggle against it. It knows nothing of your triumphs or strength. As we talked, I began realizing what would be one of the hardest lessons about my cancer. Randomness.

One person gets it, and one person doesn't. One person lives, and one person dies. Despite your treatment, personal character, or how hard you fight, the dice roll and come up as they will. We have our illusions about control. In truth, there are many things we do have control over. But there are easily as many things that leave us helpless. Our control is only over how we face them.

That morning, I stopped in the hospital's gift shop in the lobby for gum or batteries for my Discman or something like that. I heard the woman behind the counter say something about how the towers were gone. I thought, "Yeah, right." The idea was impossible to fathom. I left the hospital and caught the subway and then the streetcar home.

That morning, I watched the footage on every channel for hours. The planes hit the towers again and again in slow motion. The towers collapsed. The debris cloud raced through the streets as people ran.

And I felt nothing.

In my head, I knew how horrible it was, the tragedy of those lives lost in those few hours. But I didn't feel it. I didn't have any revulsion at humans who could perpetrate such an atrocity. I didn't have any grief for the families left behind. My soul didn't cry out in rage. I watched and thought how much it looked like special effects. It looked exactly as how I imagined a movie about it would look. My every reaction was detached and intellectual. I was watching a turning point in history as if it was nothing more than a summer blockbuster. Eleanor worried for her cousins who lived in New York. At one point, Gordon gasped, "Louise!" He then ran upstairs to try calling a friend preparing for her Broadway debut. I sat on the couch and watched, calm and unmoved.

When I spoke to Jon the next month, I told him about feeling somewhat ashamed that there was nothing except a void where the reasonable and expected emotions should have been. He told me I wasn't the first person to sit in that chair and express that feeling. He had heard it more than once. He said, "You've all already had your own personal September 11." I didn't know if I was going to live. I had fought against the disease and given it my leg as a blood sacrifice. I had been given another round of horror in return. I couldn't believe in a future. Every breath and moment was an effort just to keep moving. And there was only more to come. They were going to cut my chest open, pry my rib cage apart, and cut pieces out of the organs I was barely forcing to breathe some days. They couldn't give me a guarantee that I wouldn't have to go through it more than once.

The first fuel-bloated plane hit my life when I was first diagnosed. Unlike that morning in New York, it had taken eighteen months for the second plane to hit.

What disturbed me most in that new post-September 11 world was the attitude that the stable, white picket fence life in the suburbs as well as the warm, nuclear family and prosperous yuppie life should somehow have protected people from tragedy. The American Dream should have shielded the "greatest country in the world" from sorrow and grief. On a purely personal level, there was an attitude that only heterosexuals lost loved ones on that terrible day. In my new world of grief and loss of all I had been, I knew all too well that sorrow and tragedy are no respecters of anything. They visit all, and the people who lost their lives on that day and those who were left behind were not alone in their sudden, shattering pain.

The day after the towers fell, I reported to the hospital again for my fourth cycle of chemo. The routine was the same except for one thing. Because I had been vomiting the last two cycles, Dr. Blackstein substituted another antinauseant for the Granesitron. I don't remember what it was called, but I remember far too vividly the result of the change. The vomiting came on like a force nine gale, despite nothing being in my stomach. I vomited clear bile twice as forcefully, twice as long, and twice as often. When it seemed like I couldn't take it any longer, like my body would invert itself in it's desperation to expel the toxic brew, it was time for another dose of antinauseant. It was then back to the Granesitron. Finally, around noon on that fourth vomitous Thursday, it stopped. I barely moved for the rest of the day, weak from the nausea, effort, and relief. I don't think I did much else for the rest of my stay nor the weekend at home.

If I remember anything from those fifteen weeks of chemotherapy, it's the overwhelming sensation of just struggling to endure, holding on to the idea that the horrible sickness was worthwhile. I don't think I really lived during that time. I just existed. I stopped being a person and became a vessel. I was a battleground assaulted on one front by the sarcoma and chemotherapy on the other. My body was the scorched earth, the poisoned waters, and the scarred, blackened landscape. My hair was gone. (I finally gave up and plucked the last few hairs of my eyebrows.) My skin was pale and yellowish. I gained thirteen pounds from fluid retention, leaving me bloated and slow on top of my weakness. Several people said I looked good. I could only think, "Compared to what?!" How cadaverous and battered had they expected me to look if this was looking good? I can officially tell you that no one except Whoopi Goldberg looks good without eyebrows.

One Saturday, in the time between that cycle and the next, I was sitting in the front window of the Tango Palace reading a book that Kim had left for me, a collection of the Sandman comic books written by Neil Gaiman. On the street, I saw a man with a camera peering in and lining up various shots. He eventually came in and said he needed a photo of someone reading in a café for a Tourism Ontario brochure. He asked if I minded if he took my picture. Despite how foul I felt and worse and how I felt I looked, I said yes. I remember feeling nothing more than a weary resignation. Protesting or explaining would take too much effort. As Margot put it when I told her the story, "I am so not vain anymore!"

Despite the loss of vanity, dignity, and the sanctity of my body and despite the utter powerlessness and total lack of control over my destiny (or maybe even because of all of these things), I still hoped. But hope can be double-edged. It can keep us strong against woes and trials that would otherwise overwhelm us. If we hope for something we can't reasonably expect, the dashing of that hope can be devastating and wound us even more deeply. Somewhere in those glowing reports of the efficacy of the chemo, my mind somehow went back to that place where there would be no need for surgery because the chemo would destroy my tumours completely. There would be no need for the general anaesthetic, the bone saws, or the sutures. Once again, I allowed myself to hope that the gods would spare me.

On the eve before my last cycle of chemotherapy, I barely slept. For the last four cycles, I had gone to bed nervous, coasting to sleep while fighting dread. Somehow, I thought it would be easier that last time. The knowledge it was the last time would give me peace of mind. After this last time, there would be no more vomiting or bone-crushing fatigue. My body would begin to repair the damage done by the drugs. There would be no more antibiotics or blood work in between cycles of poison. I should have been excited, pleased, or something. But I lay there in the dark, collapsed in on myself with anxiety as if the coming three days were something new and horrible I had no foreknowledge of. It was like I was traipsing into the unknown instead of bringing the whole fifteen-week ordeal to a close.

The next morning, October 3, Dr. Blackstein confirmed the dramatically positive response to the protocol and informed me how much the tumours had shrunk. He was going ahead and asking Dr. Johnston to book a surgery date. My face and spirits fell. My vain hope for a reprieve was dashed. I was headed for the operating table once again.

Seeing my reaction, he asked why "I looked like I'd lost my best friend." I told him what I had hoped for. In the most kindly tone I think I ever heard him use, he explained the surgery was necessary. I knew he was right. Every tool had to be used to remove as much of the cancer as possible. Even a single cell could start it all over again. He said the average number of times this surgery had to be done was two point two. Any tumours too small to be seen or felt would be missed and would continue growing. There was still no guarantee that this would end it.

The one bright side of that last cycle was that Dr. Blackstein agreed to double my dose of Granesitron, giving it to me twice a day rather than once. It did the trick. There was no vomiting that last time. I have no words to describe what a relief that was. Between my exhaustion from not sleeping and the soporific effect of the antinauseant, I got into bed and promptly slept. I slept through the Doxo and woke at one point to find Gordon sitting by the bed, reading. I think that is one of the safest feelings in the world, being watched over while you sleep. It may have been the safest I had felt in months.

Late that day around dinnertime, I heard Dr. Blackstein talking to a woman about her son in the cubicle across from mine. This young man had, not one, but two primary tumours with metastases in his lungs. His chances would have been slim with one primary, but the presence of the second primary reduced his chances of even surviving to less than 10 percent. I remember his mother sounded so desperately grateful that they were even trying to save him.

My path through cancer was inhabited with people like this, and they always seemed to show up when my determination was flagging. At those times, I always crossed paths with someone who probably wasn't going to make it, whose situation was worse than mine. Despite the horrors visited on me (the pain, humiliations, and despair), it seemed likely I would survive.

After that final skirmish of chemical warfare, after the last round of Cipro and blood work, another of those forced lulls came while my body and immune system recovered enough to allow me to heal from the coming surgery. My white blood cells began recovering and replacing themselves. Within a few weeks, my hair began slowly growing back.

As before, when the recovery period drew to a close, about a week or so before the surgery, I would go for a preadmission appointment to speed the process of entering the hospital on the day. There would also be a brain and abdominal CT and a bone scan (deep imaging), once again augmented by the injection of a contrast medium into my veins to highlight any potential problems. It was called a full metastatic workup, and it frightened me anew as I got the distinct impression from Dr. Johnston that the surgery would not proceed if the scans showed any signs of further metastasis. I read the subtext as, "If anything shows up, why bother?" Dr. Satok reassured me it would only mean the treatment plan would change. My nerves settled as much as possible. Now I was heading into at least vaguely familiar territory. I knew surgery and recovery.

When the preadmission at Toronto General came, it was more comprehensive than it had been at Mount Sinai. It took more than three hours. I again had my medical history and blood taken. I met the head thoracic nurse. I was given a wrapped betadine scrub sponge to wash with on the morning before the surgery. They also gave me a sky blue gizmo called an incentive respirometer. One end of a tube goes in your mouth. In the chamber, a plastic ball rises as you inhale, like one off those carnival strength tests where you hammer a trigger to ring a bell. By adjusting the resistance on the gauge, you make it easier or harder. They told me I would need to breathe deeply and cough a great deal after the surgery to keep my lungs clear, bracing my broken sternum with my arms as I did. I was given a tour of the step-down unit, a special eight-bed ward where I would spend the first night or two being monitored. The respiratory physiotherapist walked me around the floor several times while measuring my oxygen saturation. I was given pamphlets and papers on pre- and postoperative care. I went for X-rays. I met the anaesthetist, and he briefed me on the anaesthetic and postoperative pain control.

I would have another epidural, but higher up my spine. Finally, I was done. I only had to show up on November 8.

My sister Jennifer would be the head cheerleader this time, arriving a few days before the surgery to stand guard in the waiting room. As before with Linda, we had a chance to relax and spend some time together. My parents, Linda, and her partner Alex were in England and had been for most of my course of chemo. They would not return until after the surgery. I had a knack for getting sick only when they were on vacation. Jennifer and I went to the Beaches, and I introduced her to the girls. We shopped. Honestly, that woman has the most uncanny knack for shopping. If there is a deal to be found, she'll find it. She bought me a fleece, zip-front sweater because I realized I would not be able to pull a T-shirt or sweater over my head once I was home from the surgery. It would be buttoned and zip-front clothes for me for the six weeks of recovery.

As it had been with Linda, that day or so was just a distraction. It was white noise to drown out the sound of fear. However, when we returned to the apartment, there was a message waiting for me from Dr. Johnston's secretary, Frances. The radiologist who had evaluated my brain CT had "seen something." (Again with that vague phrase!) I had been scheduled for an MRI of my head the next morning at Princess Margaret, an hour or so before I was due at Toronto General.

On top of this new surgery in a hospital I didn't know with a whole new set of recovery difficulties, there was suddenly the possibility of a brain tumour. Would they even go ahead with the surgery? Would this be the final curtain, the tumour that would be impossible to treat? Wasn't I frightened enough that day?

In the months after that recurrence, I realized, after the chemo and the surgery were over and the long emotional grief and healing was underway, that was, in many ways, the hardest part.

I had endured the initial trauma and treatment, the leg surgery, and the long, brutal course of retraining my body needed to imitate the things it used to be able to do. Just as I had gained some handle on my body, I had gone through it all again but in a completely different way. The illness, treatment, and surgery were different. The whole arena, playing field and game pieces, had been unfamiliar. On the eve of my second surgery, another wild card was thrown on the table, one that could have meant another unfamiliar game.

As I had done for the first surgery, I had power of attorney documents drawn up. This time, I gave Jennifer the power to make decisions if necessary.

Once again, I slept only fitfully the night before the surgery. I lay in the dark with my stomach churning until I grew too exhausted to not sleep. Until recently, I didn't know that Jennifer barely made it to turn the lights out before she fell apart at the thought of another trial ahead. She's a softy, but she was solid in my presence. When I needed her to be the one that was okay, she was.

In the morning, I showered with the special disinfecting sponge, covering myself in the rust-coloured lather. There was little talk as we prepared to leave. There were no expressions of anything we might be feeling. We just went through the motions, like going to the hospital to be cut open was normal. I guess it was in my new world.

We took a cab to Princess Margaret, which, except for the overtaxed medical imaging department, was deserted at that early hour. Jennifer knitted while I watched the clock and the minutes tick by, making us late. Even when I'm headed for a date to have my ribs split open, I don't want to be late.

As the conversation turned to the absurdities of not being able to take knitting needles onto a plane in the post-9/11 world, I was called in. There were the same questions about working with metal, except now a part of my body was metal. There was the same punishing sound from the same immense machine. This time, it was centred around my head, which was held steady by a tight, cagelike brace. Again, it was good I was not claustrophobic.

It was over, and we walked to Toronto General for my next appointment with the scalpel. When we arrived, Kerry was there, having arrived on time and not knowing we would be late. In the months since he had moved out and built his new life, in the face of my recurrence and treatment, we had found a way to become friends again. All of the anger I felt melted away. It just didn't matter anymore. That's how I have found it is with anger. Keeping it for a long period requires energy and commitment. All of my energy was directed elsewhere at fighting the disease, recovering from the disease, or fighting the disease again and staying alive. I released the things I had done wrong and let go of the things I felt he had done wrong. We were at last free to just be friends and relish the things we had in common. (It's funny. When I showed the first draft of this book to friends who knew us both, one said I had been too hard on him. Another said I let him off too easily.)

At the hospital that morning, I was given a bag to put my clothes in. I was taken to a waiting room where I was weighed and given a hospital gown. Then my chest was shaved. The remaining hair I had not lost and the hair that had just begun growing back was clipped down to stubble. (They don't blade shave any-more because it only irritates the skin and increases the chance of infection.) After a short wait, I was taken to the operating room's anteroom. It was both a parking lot and staging area where we waited to be whisked to our respective operating rooms. The ritual litany was repeated. "What's your date of birth?" "Do you have any allergies?" (I've grown so tired of answering those questions that I'm tempted to put the answers on flash cards.) After handing off my glasses, I was off again.

Again, the operating room was cold and bright, like those midwinter days when there are no clouds in the sky and the sunlight is sharp and hard like glass. All around were machines, trays of instruments, and masked, gowned figures bustling at their preparations. It's an odd sensation with these faceless, shapeless, sexless (until they speak) people talking in kind, efficient tones.

One of them (I think it was the anaesthetist) put in an IV and the epidural. He then administered something that made the world soft and blurry.

My understanding of what happened next is this. Once properly anaesthetized, I was intubated with a special tube that allowed them to deflate each lung separately. While they were working on one lung, the other did the work. (Only Jennifer's daughter, Erin, posed the question of how a surgeon works on your lungs when you need them to breathe.) An incision was made in my chest, exposing my sternum, which was then sawed through. (More power tools again.) With a rib spreader, they exposed my chest cavity and lungs. The first was deflated, and the tumours were identified. Surprisingly, I later discovered this was done partially by feel and this tactile examination could often tell more than a CT scan. Once located, the tumours were removed. Small conical sections of lung tissue around them were taken, and the incisions were sutured closed. The lung was then reinflated, and the procedure was repeated on the other lung. The severed edges of my sternum were then brought together and wired tightly. Two drainage tubes were inserted in the chest cavity through two small incisions below my ribs. The incision in my chest was sutured closed. (I might add it was beautifully done because not a stitch was visible.) I was extubated and sent to the step-down unit.

When I awoke, I was once again Borg boy. I had two drain tubes, a Foley catheter, an IV line, an arterial line for drawing blood, and the epidural. But another major milestone was over.

Eighteen
Recovering Again

When I regained consciousness in the step-down unit, I was surprisingly lucid, surprisingly quickly.

The unit itself is rectangular with two beds at each end and four along the long wall. A nurse's station is between two doors on the other long wall. Separated by curtains, each bed bears a patient fresh from surgery on their chest and lungs.

The day-and-a-half I was in the step-down unit was fraught with drama, none of it mine. One older man refused to sit still, constantly trying to get out of bed or eat or drink something despite the nasalgastric tube feeding him. Another man, perhaps in his fifties or sixties, woke from his anaesthesia in a state of acute paranoia. (It is apparently something that sometimes happens with men that age.) As soon as he could speak, he began accusing the doctors, nurses, and even his wife of some great conspiracy. As he raved at them, trying to pull the tubes from his body, security had to be called to keep him from hurting himself.

I seemed to be doing fine. Jennifer and Gordon were there when I woke and said Dr. Johnston had spoken to them and had said all had gone well. As soon as I was lucid enough to understand him, he actually came to see me. The surgery had lasted around two-and-a-half hours, and I had not lost much lung tissue. When the respiratory physiotherapist came around and measured my oxygen saturation, it was well into the midnineties.

The next day, the nurse helped me into another of those high, padded walkers and walked me around the floor, tiring me out. When I returned to my bed, I splinted my chest with my arms and coughed up bloody mucus, clearing away the debris the surgery left.

Later that first full day, they moved me from the step-down unit to a four-bed room where I would recover for the next three days. I remember the man in the bed across from mine, a stick-thin Asian man who seemed ancient. Every time he went to the washroom, his gown would open and expose his wrinkled, leathery bottom for all to see. Other than that, I remember resting and coughing, watching TV, and being visited. I remember being woken in the night for pills. There were more blood thinners to prevent blood clots. (Intramuscular injections left my upper arms mottled with bruises.) Percocet was given when the epidural was removed. On Saturday, November 10, Sue arrived to provide the next wave of support.

All in all, it was an uneventful hospital stay. Unlike the last surgery, there were no infections or any traumas or setbacks requiring a long stay. Over the four days, I was quietly disconnected from the various tubes and lines. The most dramatic of those was the removal of the drain tubes that required two nurses to complete. I had to bear down, holding my breath while one nurse pulled what felt like a foot-and-a-half of tubing from my chest. The other nurse pulled the suture tight, closing the wound. If I breathed at the wrong time, while the hole to my chest cavity was open, air would have entered through the hole. You can imagine what it would be like to have air in the chest cavity, outside the lungs where it belongs.

I remember the epidural needle stinging when it came out and the catheter as well, but those pains were minor compared to the pain that would follow when I was released from the hospital.

The stitches from the drain tubes were removed a day after the tubes, and they sent me home with prescriptions in hand. The ensuing days passed in a haze of pain. Narcotics dulled, along with all other sensations, the pain. Bone pain is one of the worst kinds of pain there is. It's the kind of pain that takes your breath away. Your torso is the centre of your body, the root of your extremities. Every movement springs from it and is affected by it. When it is in pain, that pain radiates through your entire body. You cannot lift your arm without pain. You cannot sit or stand without pain. You cannot even turn your head. To ease the pain of my sawed and wired sternum, I began with two Percocet every three hours. (If any of you have taken Percocet, you know how strong and addictive it is. It's one of the prescription painkillers that stars often enter rehab to withdraw from.) Within the week, I could reduce that to every four hours. To maintain the schedule and adequate pain control, they told me to make sure I set my alarm for halfway through the night, exactly four hours from the previous dose. I would have to wake myself from sleep and struggle into an upright position. (It's damn difficult when you can't push yourself up. You have to pull yourself up with your muscles, mostly your abs. Even that effort strains your chest.) I opened the bottle, took the pills with water, and then levered myself back down. Of course, I could only sleep on my back because trying to sleep on my side put unbearable pressure on my rib cage.

That was my life for about four weeks as the pain eased. I took pills every four hours just to keep the pain at bay. After about a week-and-a-half (long enough to become completely habituated), I was stepped down to Tylenol 3. The entire time, I took a stool softener to fight the constipating effects of the Oxycodone and codeine. The pain eventually eased.

Dr. Johnston said I could go back to work when I felt ready as long as I stringently followed the "no lifting, pushing, or pulling" rule. I returned after two weeks for short, exhausting shifts. Once again, it was the beginnings of Christmas season, even though it was much calmer than the Eaton Centre. Unlike the previous Christmas, I was a spare, bonus body for Jen. She had hired her seasonal employees on the assumption I wouldn't be back in time. I worked for about two-and-a-half weeks before I received my early Christmas present. My family had arranged a ticket home. For the first time in years, I would spend the holidays in the house I grew up in.

I flew into Saskatoon on December 16 and spent a week seeing friends, once again confirming I had returned from that shadowy place of "not quite life" I had disappeared into. I went with Kim and Linda to see the first movie in the *Lord of the Rings* trilogy. Kim hosted a grown-up dinner party on December 22. (I remember receiving an e-mail that brimmed with pleasant surprise at the idea. It was like the thought occurred to her out of the blue one day. We are grown-ups now!) There were multiple courses and much good conversation. Linda was there, as were my old friends, Scott Blythe and Dan Sutherland. Pauline made it for a drink, and so did my dear friend, Suzanne North, and her husband, Don Buckle. Suzanne has been my writing mentor for many years, encouraging me, goading me, and keeping me aware of the fact I can indeed write.

I think what I did in that week-and-a-half in Saskatoon that was the most significant and the most meaningful was get my picture taken. In those first weeks out of the hospital after the resection of my leg, while hobbling around my apartment on crutches (I think even before I had even been outside), a thought entered my head. It was one of those thoughts that blindsides you and makes you wonder where it came from. It was a thought that seems so unlike you that it seems it must have come from someone else's brain.

I don't know if you have seen it, but there is the most amazing photo of a woman who has had a mastectomy. She is standing against a backdrop of sky. She is topless with her arms outstretched. Around the scar that marks where her breast once was, she has a twining tattoo. Her manner is so self-confident and so comfortable with who she is and how she looks that you can't help but be moved. You can't help but know what she has survived and how it has made her brave.

The foreign thought in my head that day, so strange that it seemed I had thought it in Portuguese, was that I wanted to have pictures taken like that. I wanted to do some kind of tasteful, full body nude that would show off my new scar. If you had known me then, you would have known my intense body modesty. I was never one to take off my shirt on a dance floor or on a hot summer day. Many years, I wouldn't even wear shorts. The thought I wanted to show my body off like that was completely out of character.

The instant the thought occurred to me, I knew I wanted my friend Debra Marshall to take them. While I was in Toronto, Deb was in Edmonton and then Chicago. That Christmas, she was home, having moved back a short time before. When we started e-mailing about getting together, the seed came in my mind to ask her. Across the table at City Perk, before I even had a chance to ask her, she asked me. As I described what I wanted to do, I saw her creative juices spark.

I borrowed Kim's keys, and we commandeered her apartment one afternoon while she was at work. Over the next two hours, we shot all kinds of pictures, showcasing my imperfect body in all its scarred glory. We both had ideas. I showed everything except the pink bits. We made something special that afternoon. It was a huge step in my healing to make something beautiful, to showcase my body and not hide from what had been done to it. When I received the prints, I had them scanned and posted on my Web site. They remain one of the things in my life that I am most proud of.

December 23 was dinner at Sue's place. Then I went to the house I grew up in for Christmas itself.

So much of what I remember of Christmas with my family (or any time spent with my family for that matter) has coloured what I think about comfortable social interaction in any setting. We don't squabble. We don't reject each others' ideas. We talk, laugh, and eat. We sometimes just sit comfortably in silence with each other. They shaped me and made me who I am. They made me the strong person who could and did survive cancer.

The year 2001 ended in the quiet, dark basement of my parents' home without any fanfare. I didn't want to party or be with people. The change of year wasn't something I felt the need to celebrate or rejoice in. I just wanted the year and its trials to slip away into the past. It has been that way since this ordeal began. A new year is a coming mystery, and I never know if it will bring health or another recurrence. At that moment, I know what I have left behind. It is better to scatter it on the wind like blown leaves.

When I returned to Toronto on January 3, I had a day off before returning to work. I saw Jon Hunter on January 7. There were a few social engagements in the first few weeks in January. I reconnected with a woman I went to high school with, even though I don't think we had ever spoken during those four years. The twenty-year reunion had been held the previous summer, just as my chemo had kicked into high gear and left me unable to travel. Word of my illness spread, and there were envelopes of reunion photos and a get-well card full of names I hadn't thought of in years. Rennie was one of those people. She had been living in Toronto a few years and was appearing in *Mamma Mia*. When she sent an e-mail suggesting we meet, I thought, "You never spoke to me in high school, why now?" But we had a good time. It's amazing the leveller that twenty years of life can be once you are out in the real world.

The recurring motif of the first half of that year would be grief. Unlike the Kubler-Ross neat, tidy stages, this was messy and erratic. I bounced back and forth from stage to stage, completely out of their proper order. I finally began admitting to myself that it had all been horrible, and I let those feelings out to see the light. I had lost much and gained much, but I still needed to mourn. Jon listened and guided me. Once again, I was in that state of "I'm not going to die, now what?"

My first follow-up appointment that year was February 4. From then on, I would see Dr. Blackstein every six weeks, having either a chest X-ray or a lung CT every visit. That month, as the second anniversary of my diagnosis approached, I wrote on my Web site:

Two years.

The equivalent of half a college degree spent fighting against the results of a random mutation of my cells.

Two years of hard work and of needles and blood. Of sickening, bone-deep nausea and hard radiation. Of hard work, physical and mental. Two years of just hanging on.

Here I am—radiation, physiotherapy, chemotherapy, and two major surgeries later. I'm sterile. (Not a big issue, granted, but...) I can't walk without pain or my cane. I tire more easily. The bones of my sternum still ache from being sawed apart in this last surgery. I can't go dancing. (Maybe I could flail about a bit, but, to really cut loose like I used to, not anymore.)

During it all, I managed to dredge up strength I didn't know I had. No matter how hard or unpleasant it got, I faced it. Despite the occasional freak-out, I kept on. I stayed the course. I found more inside of me than I thought was there. More emerged.

I am both less and more than I was. This new, tempered, deeply changed me doesn't quite know what comes next. I had so many thoughts about going to school or getting a new job, moving up in the world somehow.

All I can think of now is peace. I need some time to just go to work and earn a pay-cheque, to talk to people and smile and laugh, to maybe date, and, if the gods are kind, to maybe even find love again. (The old me would have said I earned some happiness and joy, that I was due. The new me knows the randomness of it all. That two years of hell is no guarantee of a great karmic turn of the wheel.)

I want to just go to bed and wake up the next morning without any thoughts of death, cancer, and pain, to just live for a little while in quiet until the next set of hurdles comes my way. We'll deal with them when the time comes. Not before.

◆   ◆   ◆

Anniversaries are powerful emotional triggers. They can bring back memories you thought you had dealt with a long time before. That's how it was for me as winter began waning that year. I was haunted and shell-shocked by what had happened to me. Several months later, Rennie said I had seemed despondent the first time we met. I thought I had been hopeful and upbeat. I know I smiled and laughed in those months. I know I joked and spent time with friends, but I don't think I really lived or felt real joy. I knew I wanted to find it again.

I discovered instant messaging and a couple new Web sites: GayCanada and GayToronto. Through these tools, I attempted to forge new connections, even though the people were often far away. I made friends with a sweet man in Brazil, Carlos Miranda. I went on a few dates. I know now that the old dysfunction (the need to have someone and not be alone) was stirring to life again. I thought I was ready to move on. If I opened the doors, someone would sooner or later walk through. I just craved sooner more than later. That was where I was when Colin McConnell entered my life.

I logged on to GayCanada one day, and there was an e-mail for me from Colin. He had read my profile, and it sparked his interest. Then he read my Web site and learned of my battle against cancer. He told me he knew right then that he had to get to know me. I thought that was nice of him, but I didn't really expect anything to come of it. He was living in Red Deer, Alberta, at the time.

That kind of interest is seductive. For someone in the position I was in, still so damaged from all that had happened, it was a lifeline. Here was someone who knew instantly he wanted to be a part of my life somehow. What difference did distance make? You hear stories every day of people who meet online. Someone then moves, and they begin a life together. It's a reality of the new millennium.

Colin and I exchanged e-mails and then began talking on the phone—intense, deeply real conversations that lasted hours. We explored each other over the phone. One day, he said it was like the Victorian era. Because we couldn't rush to bed or into anything because of the distance, we had to court each other. He told me he was in Red Deer because he was helping his sister raise her children after the sudden death of her husband. How do you not fall in love with that? He had been thinking about leaving Red Deer. Toronto was a possibility.

I thought it was all somehow insane. No one falls in love that way. But, more than one person asked, "Why not?" Why couldn't two people fall in love that way? I honestly think they were right. Love can grow in a situation like that. But, in the end, the broken link would turn out to be me.

Colin had vacation time coming, and we arranged for him to come and visit to test what we had begun to feel. We would get to know each other in person. He would scout the work situation. (He was a hairstylist.) He would see if it was a city he wanted to live in.

The day he was due to arrive, April 16, actor Robert Urich died after a long battle with cancer, specifically synovial sarcoma. He was the only other person I have known of that had the same disease as me. And now he was dead. Was that what I had to look forward to? Was that to be my fate? It had already recurred once. My future was suddenly cast in doubt again. Like Sandra Sprecker's father so many years before, now one person suddenly represented so much more. Now, synovial sarcoma equalled death. I was contemplating a future with Colin, yet I was suddenly feeling like I had no future.

The day Colin arrived, I traipsed out to the airport to meet him. (Before that, I never knew you could TTC from my place all the way to the airport!) We spent ten days together and had a lovely time. The first tentative steps toward a plan were made. He explored the area while I was working. Then it was time for him to leave, and we went back to talking on the phone and sending e-mails.

For me, something changed. I'm not excusing or justifying myself, just reporting how I felt. Where once our exchanges had been saturated with content, we seemed to be reduced to "Just wanted to tell you I love you." The love I had wanted to find was now out of reach again. I had wanted to have someone in my life, but I seemed to only have a theory of love.

To tell the truth, I was still broken inside. The rough edges were still grinding against each other. The thought of this man uprooting his life and leaving his family behind for me was too much for me to bear. I had borne this horrible disease and struggled to carry my own life in my hands. Now I was suddenly carrying the responsibility for his life. I couldn't take it. I wasn't ready for it. It was, in many ways, so like me. I so often crave that kind of love and have no idea what to do with it when it comes. Then I met someone else.

Never before did I start a new relationship before the one I was in ended and never since. Like it happens with so many other people, Dawson and I just began chatting and had an initial meeting over coffee. I was attracted to him right away. He's the type that just comes at you with this intense energy and sense of fun. He was playful and intelligent. Originally from Turkey, he had only been in the country for less than a year when we met. One night, while talking on the phone, we were watching a documentary on the Discovery Channel about Turkey. He described the places we were watching. At one point he said, without any self-pity in that ebullient way he had, "I miss my country!"

He invited me over for dinner, and I stayed until Saturday morning, coming home to a forlorn e-mail from Colin. I did the only thing I could do and owned up to what had happened, explaining the reasons as best I could. I beat myself up well and truly that weekend. Despite how it had happened, I knew the decision was the right one, and that was part of what hurt the most. I hadn't seen it for what it was and had allowed my own emotional turmoil to hurt someone else.

Where Colin was ready to remake his life in my image, Dawson was refreshingly not. He was not "out" at work or to his Turkish friends, even though he was happily out to himself. Although my already slightly bent rule about dating men in the closet was still in place, I tried my best to understand. He was from another culture and half a world away from his family. His Turkish friends were a link to his home and part of a very different world with very different views on homosexuality. Maybe I just let it slide because I wanted him. I don't really know. But he was a tonic for me. He wasn't looking to move in with anyone or settle down. He wanted a boyfriend, not a husband. In my emotional state at the time, I was happy to oblige. I would work my shift at the store, hop on the streetcar to Dawson's place, and spend the night. I brought him to the store. He met Sandra Hutchinson, who pronounced him "hot" and loved his cologne.

In many ways, he was the perfect summer fling. But summer ends. Eventually, the feeling there was no future in store for me would fade. My need for space and freedom would ease, and I would find myself in exactly the opposite position I had been with Colin. I would want to settle down again and be with someone who didn't want what I wanted.

Nineteen
Summer and Change

That summer would be one of calm and stability. When the merger between Indigo and Chapters took place, the two women who knew me as well as my abilities and strengths left the company in the restructuring. I was in a position with no allies above me. I had been offered the promotion at Store #3 by my then-regional manager, who believed in me and my skills. Now, she and her replacement, who had moved me to Store #585, were both gone.

When I returned from my chemo and surgery, the store regulars again embraced me and welcomed me back. Linda Livingstone, a model/actress and one of the most beautiful, older women I have ever seen, possessed a generous, caring spirit. Mrs. Kelly came in every week for her Harlequin romances. Mrs. Iverson hugged me the first time she saw me back, barely coming up to my chest. Lise O'Sullivan was a firecracker with a mouth like a longshoreman, but she had a kind soul underneath. Unlike my first time away, I returned to someplace safe.

I took over our special orders, streamlining and monitoring the process and making some people happy in the process. One was so happy that he wrote an e-mail to our customer service manager about me. I made sure our new regional manager knew about it.

I loved the store and the company in those days, but it was tiring and hard on my leg. On top of that, customer service jobs are never paid as well as they should be. Indigo paid well in terms of industry standards, but industry standard doesn't pay good retail people enough. I was struggling against debt incurred when Kerry and I split up as well as when I was ill. I knew I would eventually have to find a more lucrative job if I ever wanted to get ahead.

Jen (bless her heart) made sure Mark, the regional manager, knew I had been in management and how happy she had been those months I was there. He took me aside one day to ask about my plans. I wanted to advance in the company in some way, but I needed to get off the sales floor. I wanted to explore options in our home office if they came up. He suggested I keep up on the job postings and said he would stay in my corner when the time came.

There was a management change that summer. Jen wanted to be closer to home and needed a change. She switched places with another manager. It was a tough transition for everyone with differing expectations and methods of working. Things eased eventually, but the air was always a bit strained.

One day, a job posting came up at our support office for our SOS (store operations support) hotline. We often called them for issues relating to our loyalty card program or with questions about promotions and such. We all felt we knew the people on the other end, even though we had never met them. It wasn't exactly what I wanted to do. My first, dream choices were procurement or marketing, but there was no time to stop and think. The posting arrived on Thursday, and the deadline for applying was Monday. If there was even a chance I wanted it, I had to apply now and think later. We spent the next few days madly getting the appropriate forms and faxing them to the appropriate place.

The round of checkups continued. I lived my life in those six-week chunks with apprehension growing each time the appointment approached. Each time, things were fine, and my apprehension began slowly easing. Maybe this cancer didn't equate with death after all. Maybe there was a vague hope for a future after all.

◆　　　◆　　　◆

08*13*02

Today was my latest checkup. It was all clear without any signs the cancer had returned. I got another six-week reprieve. It would be another six weeks before I have to face that nagging fear again. I have another six weeks to pretend that everything is normal.

Granted, the fear is lessening each time. Every time I go, I feel more relaxed and more certain it will be fine and there will be no more cancer.

Even that is a bit frightening, the possibility of being lulled into a false sense of security, only to be slammed back to earth really hard at a later date. There's this feeling I must stay vigilant and gird my strength, just in case. I remember around the anniversary of the discovery of the cancer in my lungs suddenly having no idea how I had done it or how I had fought it. How I had won. That was terrifying because I had no idea how I would do it again if I had to. As time passed, I remembered the techniques. I remembered the love and strength showered on me by those who love me and those who took care of me. I remembered what I found inside me that made me able to fight. It felt good to have those weapons back in my arsenal—just in case.

Believe me, if I have any say in the matter, I am not doing this again. Today, I'm one small step closer to putting this behind me for good.

◆　　　◆　　　◆

The day after I wrote that, the gamble of my application worked. I received a call for an interview for the hotline job. It was another small, hopeful gift that moved me further along the path of healing.

◆　　　◆　　　◆

08*14*02

I have an interview for the job I applied for! It's an internal position, an operator for the store hotline. I will be off my feet. I think the pay is better, and it will get me closer to a job at the home office. I'd eventually like something in marketing or procurement, and this will at least put me on the radar, make me known to the people in the positions to make that happen. When you're as far away from everything as I am out in the Beaches, you practically don't exist to the people who are guiding the direction of the company.

But, gods, the prospect of another job interview with those awful, HR questions! "Tell me about a time when you showed leadership ability… Tell me about a time when you resolved a conflict with a coworker." It's enough to freeze the blood! I actually went for a job as a call centre worker for Visa last summer between bouts of cancer. I was only told afterwards that they weren't offering me the job because they didn't think I could handle the stress. (?!?!?) Yah, okay sure, fine! Whatever those little test questions say, dude!

I'm a little apprehensive because the job will be with a new version of the hotline, combining the tech support and store operations functions again. I mean, I know my way around a computer, but I'm self-taught mostly. When it comes to hardware issues, I'm screwed. But, when all else fails, bluff and refer the caller to someone who knows! I think most of this kind of thing is knowing who to properly pass the problem along to. I'm damn good at that!

So, we'll see. When Todd called, he sounded eager to interview me for the job, so I guess that's a good sign. Now all I have to do is not get my hopes up.

◆　　　◆　　　◆

I felt good about the place as soon as I walked into 82 Peter Street. I liked Todd and Bozana, the two people I would be working with. As soon as I walked into that room, I knew I wanted the job. I had no idea if I could do it or if I was up to the change, but I knew I wanted to find out. I was interviewed for the job by Todd (a walking encyclopaedia of company processes) and Valerie Loncar, who would be the new head of the unified tech and operations hotline. Valerie is petite and elfin with her cropped, spiky hair, but there's steel under there. She knows what she's doing and what she expects of you. Even then, I felt the interview went well.

◆   ◆   ◆

08*20*02

I had my interview today for the hotline job. I'm not sure. I can never tell about these things. I think it went well. Thankfully, it was almost all questions like, "How would you deal with…What would you do if…" I find those much easier to answer than those where you have to come up with some concrete example of your past behaviour to illustrate your perfect suitability for the position.

Todd and Valerie both seemed pleased with my responses and my personality. Hopefully, all of the other candidates will be total duds. It's a nice office space with lots of light and nice workstations. The chair was a religious experience! It was one of those Sharper Image-esque, black, mesh-backed things with more adjustments and knobs than I'd know what to do with! The chair was what really sold me.

So, it's done. I survived it, and I think I managed to get across my suitability for the job. Now it's up to them. And I won't stew about it…much.

◆   ◆   ◆

My emotional life, on the other hand, was not so satisfying. Dawson and I continued our pattern. Our relationship played out at his place. We saw each other for three months. He never once stayed at my place. In that time, we never grew and progressed. Part of that was just the nature of our schedule. I was working mostly afternoon to evening shifts, while he was working a normal morning to afternoon workday. The evenings and nights were the only times we had together. His weekends were spent with his circle of Turkish friends, who would never even know I existed. The freedom and lack of constraint that had so appealed began chafing.

◆   ◆   ◆

Funk…and not in a groovy, "dance your ass" off sort of way. It's more that, blue, not quite satisfied, kind of way. I'm tired of the dating merry-go-round. It just seems kind of pathetic to be still doing this in the last six months before my fortieth birthday. It's not glamourous and Sex and the City. *It's just kind of annoying.*

I'm seeing a guy who is wonderful, but he can't offer me anything more than once a week. He never let me meet any of his friends because he's in the closet. I swore I'd never do that again, but I broke the rule for him. I've met a couple of nice guys. There's the stand-up comedian who two different people have told me sets off their gaydar, yet he's never been anything but friendly or indicated anything about his orientation. There was the gorgeous African-Canadian guy who seemed interested and was pumping a mutual friend for information about me, but he hasn't called. (Yes, he has my number!)

All of it seems incredibly banal compared to the depth of tragedy and misery of the last few years of my life, but I think that's part of how you know your life is healing. It's no longer about vomiting, hair loss, or "Am I going to survive this?" It's just about why can't I find a nice boyfriend who isn't damaged or in the closet?

My feelings were stunted and shut down for so long. Out of sheer self-preservation, I barely let myself feel anything during the illness. I closed the pain, humiliation, indignities, and utter grief at losing my able-bodied self just to get through the next physio appointment or the next round of chemo. It was the only way I could endure it. Then, in the first months after it was all over, the grief, pain, loss, and sadness seemed to be all I could feel. A guy who didn't want to settle down and get hitched was perfect.

I didn't know if I had a future, so why plan for one? Now I've been doing well for long enough to feel like it might actually last a while, if not (knock wood and cross your fingers) for good. I want to build a future again. The job would be part of it, and the boyfriend thing would be a part of it as well. I guess this funk has a groove of its own after all.

◆   ◆   ◆

As so often happens with me, I just woke up one day and had to put a stop to it. I wasn't happy and didn't believe I would be happy at that time. Once again, I didn't handle it well. I broke up with him via e-mail. It was pretty pathetic. In retrospect, I realize I gave up too soon. If I had given it time and expressed what I needed, we might have had a chance. Maybe not. But I didn't give it a chance.

Luckily, he is a friend to this day, and we always enjoy it when we see each other. But, once again, I was deep in the dating quagmire.

◆   ◆   ◆

08*25*02

Have you ever left a job and had to write one of those "Please tell us why you are leaving this position" forms? Wouldn't it be nice if you could do that with dates? "Please tell us why you said you'd call and didn't... Please tell us why you seemed so very interested but never acted on it?"

I mean, I'm just as bad. Where is that line where you owe the person some explanation if you decide that something about your interaction with them isn't working for you? Why aren't there classes in this stuff? Better yet, why isn't there a service you could use to spare yourself and the other person emotional mess?

"Hello, is this Arthur? This is Eros Termination Services. We are calling to inform you that Stephen King has decided to end his affiliation on the grounds of differing expectations of the nature of the relationship. He has filed a friendship bid, and you have two weeks to file for friendship termination if you wish. I'll leave you my number and fax if you decide to file through us. Your case reference number is Q55-68-321. Have a nice day!"

Now that would be useful!

◆   ◆   ◆

08*26*02

I was all set to write a rant about the big lie that is "I'll call you," which so often means "I won't call you" or "I might call you, if I have nothing better to do." Then the person who hadn't called me did call and had a good reason for not calling me when he said he would.

None of which actually changes what a big lie "I'll call you" really is, but, without the righteous wrath fuelling it, my heart wouldn't be in it.

I'm extra-sensitive to it all right now. I get in these phases where I really want someone in my life, and I jones for it really badly. Then I try too hard and give my number to men I'm attracted to that I think might possibly be attracted to me. The Blitzkrieg approach rarely yields anything except me sitting by the phone upset because the man I gave my number to barely a day before hasn't called yet!

I mean really! I've faced down aggressive cancer, but the prospect of datelessness makes my blood run cold! How messed up is that!

◆   ◆   ◆

Then, the call I had been waiting for came.

◆   ◆   ◆

08*28*02

I get home from coffee at the Tango Palace this afternoon, and there's a message from one of my coworkers that the woman who interviewed me for the job had called looking for me. I called her office and left a voice mail, but I didn't hear back.

So, I'm left sitting here on tenterhooks waiting to find out whether I got the job or not! I hate waiting at the best of times, but now? I'm stuck in this feeling of "Damned if I do and damned if I don't." If I don't get the job, I'm going to be upset because I want it. If I do get the job, I'm going to be upset because I don't want to leave an environment where I'm happy.

On some level, this store is intimately bound up with my illness. I came there in my first recovery period. I got sick for the second time there and recovered again, all while being a part of that environment and neighbourhood. My customers inquired after me and made me welcome when I returned.

Now, for the first time, I feel like I have a future again, like my life isn't about illness and recovery. This job might be a new start, a new place to be in a new (hopefully) disease-free future, that is, if I get it!

Either way, I'm gaining and losing. Either way, it isn't going to be easy, and I don't really know what I'm hoping for right now. I guess I won't know until I get it.

◆   ◆   ◆

Valerie offered me the job. The salary was better. More than that, it was a promotion, a chance to move up and bring something fresh and new into my life. It was something new that wasn't about my disease. When she told me, there wasn't any doubt in my mind. I knew then that I did want it. My new manager asked if I could stay until after Labour Day when he returned from vacation. He and Valerie worked out my start date, and the die was cast.

I said my good-bye to the staff and the customers I cared about. On September 16, I began my new job, a newly christened business support analyst instead of hotline operator. At times, the transition was a difficult one. I was using mental muscles I hadn't used before. There were new computer programs and new procedures to learn. I was no longer working face-to-face with people. The only contact I had was over the phone or e-mail, but I was happy in the new place and with the new people. I learned.

Just as I was beginning to fit in, feel comfortable in my new position, and feel like it all was the right place to be, the bottom fell out again. When I reported to Dr. Blackstein on October 8, I discovered the CT I had the week before had flagged another nodule in one of my lungs.

Twenty
Three on a Match

When Dr. Blackstein told me, I sat shocked, but I was already putting on the face. There was a definite upside this time. There would be no more chemo. I would be booked straight into surgery, as soon as was possible. Quite possibly, it would even happen before Christmas.

He looked at me and asked if I was okay. Out of habit, I said yes. He said it was okay to not be okay. That time, I wasn't okay. In fact, I was nowhere close. For the first time since the whole ordeal had begun, there was bitterness. I had been angry and sad, but this was something new, something longer lasting. Once again, I had been strong and had worked hard to rebuild my life and move on. I had begun a new phase of my life. Instead of being rewarded with health or, at the very least, being left alone, I was being punished again.

The next day, I told my immediate teammates, Todd and Bozana. Valerie was out of the office that day, so I told our team lead, Michel. They were instantly supportive. When I spoke to Valerie the next day, she let me know the whole team was behind me.

An irrational guilt came with the bitterness. If the surgery happened before Christmas, I would be leaving them shorthanded during the busiest time of the year. Valerie had trusted me with this responsibility and had chosen me to be a part of her team, and I was about to let them down when they needed me the most. When I expressed this feeling, they quite rightly looked at me as if I was mad. But I couldn't help it. Deep down, I felt responsible, as if it was somehow my fault. I felt I should have warned her that this possibility existed, even though my history must have been known at the time she hired me.

Not surprisingly, my anxiety levels peaked during that time. Jon Hunter had given me a prescription for Ativan when I started having sleep problems. I was soon taking it during the day when I found myself having an anxiety attack at work. I almost broke down and cried with my back to the room. The Ativan helped in those moments of awful panic. You don't know how much stress you are under or how deep the anxiety runs until that pill kicks in and it suddenly eases, leaving only placid numbness.

When I told Dr. Satok about the tranquillizers, he suggested the possibility of something systemic rather than a spot treatment that brought me down for only short periods. I didn't consider it until the next time I was at the clinic to see Dr. Blackstein. As always, I waited for at least a couple of hours because the clinic was insanely busy. I then waited again after the clinic for blood work. It had been a long, tiring day that had started with an early morning at work. I was in the waiting room with people who were one year clear of cancer, three years clear, and five years clear. I couldn't even make it to a year. When I finally left the lab, I raced to try to catch Peter before he left. And I fell apart.

At that moment, I was willing to try anything to deal with the crushing weight of bleak anxiety on my system. Peter gave me a prescription for Citalopram, an antidepressant/antianxiety drug. I took my first pill that night.

I woke up on Wednesday in the grip of nausea I hadn't felt since my time in chemo. Because that was the day there were only two of us on the phones, I couldn't stay at home. I staggered through the day and took my next dose that night, thinking the feeling was merely an initial side effect that would pass. The next morning, it was worse. Emotionally, I was right back in the worst, most devastating time of my life. The body remembers in ways the mind can't.

I took two days off. I was shattered and barely able to move. In those two days, I slipped from pain into suffering as the walls caved in. I called Peter's office and left a message about what had happened. When he called me back, he said, "I hear I poisoned you!" We agreed I should stop the pills. As soon as the nausea began fading, my throat began to get sore. I was barely able to swallow over the weekend. I saw Peter the next week for antibiotics. Once the Citalopram was out of my system and the throat infection cleared up, I returned to my occasional use of Ativan to ease the rough days, which seemed fewer after that. I couldn't take another physical upset like that.

Around that time, I met Shayne, the third man I would date during that crazy year. As before, I met him on GayToronto. We were soon instant messaging and talking for hours on the phone. Once we met in person, it all happened fast—too fast. He was young and full of energy and desire. He was goofy, childlike, and fun to be around. It made me feel light and not weighed down by illness and fear. I wanted to be with someone in that dark time to save myself from the pain I was feeling. I let myself be swept up in it.

Far too soon, I told him I loved him. At the time, I believed it because I needed to. Instead of easing the drama, it just added to it. There was the first night I stayed over. We woke to find the guy he had been seeing on and off—the guy who had fallen for him—in the living room on the couch. There was the constant neediness, the times he kept saying something along the lines of "You're going to dump me." One time, he accused me of having someone with me when I didn't want him to come over. All was not well.

On the health front, there was something of a reprieve. The surgery would not happen until after Christmas. When the crush of pre-Christmas occurred, I would be there to fulfil my responsibilities.

The month of December passed in a flurry of support calls and e-mails. My four days off were spent recovering from the Norwalk virus. Once again, New Year's was a quiet night alone, just letting the previous year fade away.

When the surgery came, there was little warning. Like the previous time, there was preadmission to speed the process on the day. There was a sudden cancellation, and I was in the week after the phone call.

Once more, there was preadmission, and a similar routine on the morning of the surgery. Shayne stayed with me the night before and piled into the cab with Gordon and me. I was shaved again, prepped again, and sent off to another cold, bright operating room. This time, my guardians in the waiting room were three generations of boyfriends, Gordon, Kerry, and Shayne. (When the nice, little, old lady volunteering in the waiting room came around with magazines to offer them, she apparently started handing them *Sports Illustrated*. She then took a second look and offered them decorating magazines instead, sending them into gales of laughter.)

There were very few new details this time around. There was the familiar step-down unit, the epidural, the drain tubes, and the pain. New this time was a spell of vomiting when I was coming out of the anaesthetic. (It wasn't pleasant at the best of times, but it was worse with an injured rib cage.) On one day, they were manhandling me into the wheelchair to take me to X-ray, and I felt the drain tubes shifting and moving in my chest. For the next day or so before they released me, I felt a sharp pain in my side where the end of the tube grazed against muscle. When the tubes came out, they asked if some Ryerson nursing students could watch. I thought they were maybe referring to the two I had spoken to, but a ring of several ended up around the bed. I think the sight of a foot of rubber tube being pulled out of my chest left a few green.

Dr. Johnston showed a dry sense of humour the day before I was released. When I asked if I could stay until the stitches from the drain tube holes were removed, he said, "You can't do it yourself?" Then, on seeing my expression, he chuckled and said, "Look at his face!" Once again, it was home on a wave of pain and Percocet. I was back on the four-hour cycle of pills and waking in the night in agony.

Shortly after I returned home, Shayne came over with dinner on a Saturday night to watch a couple of movies on TV. He spent the entire evening stroking my hand and leg, trying to be comforting. It drove me crazy. My body hurt so much that even my skin seemed to hurt. The next day, I told him over the phone that I needed him to ease up. I needed to concentrate on healing my body and life. He said he understood, but he listened without hearing.

◆   ◆   ◆

01*27*03

"It's been a long road, getting from there to here."

It's been a long few months. Once again, I am plunged deep into cancer world with another recurrence or, rather, a remnant of my last bout. One last, small lesion is on my right lung, middle lobe. It's just a few cells missed last time. They're too small to be seen or felt, but they're growing once again.

It's been hard, this relentless pummelling of my spirit and constant destruction of my hope and to keep being sent back to a place no human being should ever have to go. But I somehow kept at it. I don't really know how. Maybe it was strength. Maybe just sheer bullheadedness. But I'm here.

They did another lung surgery two weeks ago. Dr. Johnston removed the lesion and another something he was pretty sure was scar tissue. And that hopefully is that. The indications are good. He seemed positive and optimistic.

I'm allowing myself the luxury of a bit of hope. But even hope seems strange to me after having it dashed so many times. Not to mention health! The other day, my psychiatrist said, if this is actually the end of this horrible illness, health will be a whole new thing. After all, it's been a stranger for three years.

And I'm a mess. Physically, I'm recovering nicely, but my emotions, heart, and soul are in shreds. It sometimes seems the emotional scars run deeper and more vividly than the physical ones. I met a really nice guy before Christmas, when I was buried deep in denial about the upcoming surgery, not even looking at it lurking in the background. He was sweet, fun, and totally into me, and I tumbled into it without thinking.

Then the neediness started. He kept telling me I was going to dump him. There was always this element of him wanting reassurance that I really did care for him and wasn't going to leave him. Then I went into the hospital. I was cut open, cut up, and stitched back together with tubes and catheters in every orifice. Suddenly everything was about me. I admit it. I was absorbed by the cancer vortex again. And the fun wasn't fun anymore. More than once, I told him that I needed some breathing room to heal and I didn't have much to offer. Then, one night as I lay on the couch, barely a week after the surgery and while I was in a haze of pain and pain medication, he asked me over the phone if I was having second thoughts about us.

I lost my mind and proceeded to yell at him. The bubble had burst. The feelings were gone. I couldn't reassure myself that anything would be okay. Here he was, looking to me to reassure him.

I tell myself I did the best I could and I acted with no malice, but he ended up getting hurt. And I feel nothing. I just want some peace and quiet to try to heal myself, to try to figure out what it means to be here and to still be alive.

◆   ◆   ◆

If I regret anything about those months, it's the way I treated Shayne. I knew the mess I was when we met. Granted, I didn't know how much he needed to be loved and how significant it was when I said I loved him. I wish I had been able to not hurt him, Colin, Dawson, or any of them. I wish I could have been self-aware enough to know what I was doing when I got into those relationships and been able to express what was in my heart and head. I often felt as if I should have been surrounded by traffic cones or police tape marking me as a love hazard.

In those days of healing and pills and fatigue, I voiced an opinion that I couldn't do it again. If it came back, I would let it have me. My sister Linda grew angry with me. My friend Lindsay practically went on suicide watch. Though that feeling passed, it was an important crux. In accepting that feeling, I felt empowered. I needed to feel I had a choice. After feeling helpless in the face of the disease for so long, I could choose another course if I wanted. In acknowledging I could opt to not go on, I found the strength I needed to go on.

As the pain eased and I regained my strength, I felt restless to return to work. I felt comfortable in pushing the envelope, if only slightly.

◆   ◆   ◆

01*30*03

I'm going to go into work for a couple hours this afternoon to catch up on e-mail and updates and try to get a feel for what's been happening while I was gone, that is, to ease back into real life.

I feel hesitant and unsure of the decision. I wonder if it's just that I'm unready to give up my narcotic-laced leisure or if there's something else happening. I feel almost vulnerable for some reason. I mean, I don't really know most of my coworkers that well. To disappear one day without any warning and have them find out about the cancer that way feels strange to me. I wonder what it will be like to walk into that room today. How they will act. Will they fuss or just take it in stride? How do I want them to act?

It occurred to me in the shower just now the strangeness of this shifting back and forth from the real world of bill payments, employment, and commuting into the sur-real cancer world of treatments, surgeries, and recurrences. It's been three years of fits and starts, putting life on hold to fight and then adjusting back to normalcy, only to have that normalcy shattered again and again.

Maybe that's what it is, this hesitancy. Maybe it's a reluctance, a fear of reestab-lishing normal day-to-day routines because, deep down, I just expect them to be shat-tered again later. Like some psychic equivalent of getting the bends, I need to decompress. It is like the only thing waiting for me are painful nitrogen bubbles in my bloodstream.

I guess there is hope again. It is hope that this really is the last time. But hope can be a pretty vicious mistress when she's dashed. And dashed hopes have sort of become commonplace in the last three years. If I give up hope, what kind of life have I gained?

Despite everything, I still feel like we maybe really kicked it this time. I'm still going to choose that path, despite the fears and uncertainties.

I'm still going to hope.

◆   ◆   ◆

Three weeks after getting home from the hospital, I went back to work.

◆   ◆   ◆

01*31*03

Well, I made it through my first few hours back at my desk. I waded through 212 e-mails and read up on the updates and promotions going on this month. Everyone seemed glad to see me. It was funny. David was the one who talked to me the most, and he's the quietest one there, the one who says the least.

It was okay, even though I felt a bit out of my element. It was like I didn't know what I was doing, like I'd forgotten everything. It's funny because, before I left, I felt confident. It was like I'd really gotten a handle on the job. I had worked my first Sat-urday alone and done a small bit to handle a big tech crisis.

These detours into cancer world mess with your head. They totally disconnect you from your real, everyday world. It's so easy to lose the threads of your life, the normal-cies that give you structure. I know I just have to get back on the horse, do the job, and push past this sudden insecurity, and I'll be fine. But there's still that catch of breath, that moment of fear that it's all a sham and I really don't know what I'm doing.

◆   ◆   ◆

02*02*03

Have you ever seen Breakfast at Tiffany's? *Holly Golightly talks of a phenomenon called the mean reds, something infinitely worse than the blues.*

I'm tired of rebuilding my life. I rebuilt my life here in Toronto. I rebuilt my life when Kerry and I split up. I've rebuilt my life twice since I was diagnosed with cancer. Now the prospect of doing it all again is laid in my path as I career through the last few months before turning forty.

I find I'm faced with the things I wanted out of life and wanted to accomplish. My aspirations have never been lofty, but it just isn't me. I made peace a long time ago with the fact that I would never change the world. But I wanted to find love, not just the love of friends I have in abundance, but the love of one special man who would stand at my side through the rest of my life. That seems so far out of my reach, and both are due to the prospects of wandering the streets and sorting through my own bag-gage where intimacy is concerned. I need to stop being attracted to physically or emo-tionally unavailable men. I need to stop finding the ones who are needy, insecure, still in the closet, or some other impediment from the endless list. I know what the goal is. I just don't know where the path is.

I know this feeling will pass as I get used to my job again and get used to not being sick, even if the reprieve is only temporary. But the roads are forking in front of me. I feel the pressure of time, the pressure of fewer days ahead than behind. I am leery of trying another wrong path and having to rebuild again.

◆   ◆   ◆

But rebuild I did. I kept at work, learning and making mistakes. (That, of course, I beat myself up over.) I got better at what I did. I opened myself to the possibility of meeting someone again, this time knowing I would not rush. If I was going to give my heart again, it would only be for real and for the long term. The lessons I had learned from my short time with Shayne were still burned fresh in my memory. On the rare occasions we had contact, his hurt was still pretty raw. In one instant message, he accused me of using him. I hadn't set out to, but it was hard to argue. As February ended and March began, my emotions were once again unsettled.

◆   ◆   ◆

03*03*03

I've been half a bubble off centre ever since then. I've been feeling this profound sense of disconnection. I find myself in these moods sometimes, like everything is unfamiliar. It's like I'm playing a role. I'm one of those soap characters who gets recast and the new actor doesn't look anything like the previous one.

I just get these achingly vivid sense memories of what my life was before cancer, before this litany of horrors was visited on my body and my soul. Suddenly, it's like all of this is wrong and strange. This damaged body is like a trap, something I don't belong in. These feelings aren't mine, and these hateful memories aren't mine. It all belongs to someone else. If we just touch the magic jewel at the same time, the flash of light will transfer my spirit back into my own body and my own life.

People with the best of intentions spout platitudes about how I haven't changed. I'm still me. I'm just stronger and braver than I was. Still, these days of unrelenting strangeness continue, when the weight of it hits me like a fist in the gut and I have to stop what I'm doing and breathe a moment or collapse under it all, the crests and troughs of utter strangeness and familiarity that come and go.

In the other times, it is all too familiar because I was there for it all. Despite how I might feel in those times of strangeness, I know this new life as well as this new body and soul are mine...and mine alone.

◆   ◆   ◆

03*04*03

The sense of disconnect has passed somewhat, and I realize this damaged body and this injured soul are both mine. A boundless grief at the loss and the trials I went through replace the disconnection, and I just want to sit and cry.

I hate what I've become, the hampered body and the heart and mind riddled with these hateful memories. I would erase it if I could—every treatment, every surgery, and every pain. If I could do that, I'd sacrifice the kindnesses and the wonderful people who helped me through.

If it took sacrificing all of that to be free of this, I would do it in a heartbeat just to walk unaided and unhobbled, to not feel the pain when I stand after sitting too long or when I walk and to not have these ghosts, these black memories that mar my heart like the scars mar my body.

If this was a short story or a cautionary fable, this would be the point where I would stare vehemently into the camera and swear to do anything if I could just be what I was. The devil would then appear to trade for my soul, broken though it is.

This isn't a movie, is it? I'm not some faded sitcom star groping for credibility in a disease of the week movie. No eleventh-hour happy endings or epiphanies for the protagonist. Just survival. Just a roll of the dice that comes up snake eyes if you look at it in one way and lucky sevens if you look at it in another.

◆   ◆   ◆

03*05*03

I spent the evening at the GayToronto get together tonight, the monthly face-to-face meeting. I had a great time, meeting some people I've chatted with but never seen before. I caught up with a few people I have met. My lungs ache from the cigarette smoke, and I've stayed up way too late.

It's strange to realize that not one of those people knows me from before I got sick. Not one of them has any picture of me as a whole, nonhandicapped person. None of them ever knew the precancer me. My life is becoming more and more like that. I'm looking forward to going home, just to see people who have that extra grasp of just what I lost.

There were a couple guys there, men I've chatted with who I find very attractive. When I left, I found I didn't want to be alone tonight. I wanted one of these men to come home with me. But I didn't initiate, and neither did they, assuming they were actually interested as well. I sometimes find the dark frightening. It reminds me too much of those long, fearful nights after the diagnosis, terrified at the netherworld I had entered with most of my loved ones so far away. It reminds me of those long, constantly interrupted nights of pain and fear in the hospital. I wanted the sound of someone breathing next to me in the night. I wanted someone's heartbeat against my skin.

It would merely have been sex as means to get the closeness that might have come afterward. Or it might not have.

Even though, in my time, I have been bold and blunt enough to invite sex. Asking someone to just stay with me because I'm afraid to be alone in the dark with my demons is something I've never let my guard down enough to do. I know now why I've been feeling so unsettled and plunged into my own time bomb memories. It was the end of February that I received my initial cancer diagnosis three years ago.

I turned three on the weekend.

◆   ◆   ◆

It would not be my only birthday that spring. War erupted in Iraq, and SARS erupted in Toronto. My sister, Sue, and her husband offered me a flight home on their Airmiles points. I had spoken to Valerie and Michel when I became ill again, and they were kind enough to arrange for me to use a couple weeks of my 2003 vacation time early. Once more, I would go home to see the friends I missed so much, who I had found no one like in Toronto. I was able to reconnect with some friends I had not seen in years, one of whom I just happened on in the street. Once again, I told the story to people who had no idea what had occurred. On my quiet afternoons, I found my voice again, and the fire to complete this story blazed alive in me again. I walked the familiar, yet strange streets once again, knowing I didn't want to return there to live and knowing the cool job I liked so much wasn't on those streets, in that city, or even in that province.

On April 6, we had dinner at Sue and Bill's house in Saskatoon. Linda and Alex were there, as were Suzanne, Don, and Kim. Members of my family of blood and my family of choice met for the first time. Seemingly against all odds, in the face of all that had conspired to keep me from getting there, I turned forty.

Twenty-One
Enough Already

In many ways, my fortieth year was like the years before. The aftershocks had subsided. Now it was a matter of putting everything that hadn't been broken in the quakes back in its rightful place.

It was a year of growing comfortable in my job, getting used to its new demands, and riding a series of organizational changes. We amalgamated our small operations team with the IT support team and moved into a new space in our building. I gradually developed relationships with the voices on the other ends of the phone lines and my teammates. I liked helping stores with their problems or steering them in the right direction to find the solutions they needed if I couldn't provide them. Every day, I talked to people in our stores across the country. Every day, I learned something new.

It was a year of making new friends and developing the relationships with the ones I had recently made. Nick, whom I had met the summer before, and I bonded over science fiction and comic geekery. I finally met his boyfriend, Rob. The three of us spent many an evening over coffee and sweets. Martin, who was impossibly tall, became a dear friend after a few aborted dates as he made plans to move from Kingston into Toronto. Pete was an unrequited crush that faded within weeks of meeting. We bonded over Tim Horton's coffee, telling each other things we told no one else. Bulent was the real person behind the "Dawson" I dated. I had fallen for the fiction, but I became friends with the person. Mark from work and I bonded over our mutual love of writing. Shawn from Oshawa and I regularly traded quips online. With his boyfriend, Stephen (or Namesake as I call him), he joined me for drinks at Pride.

Spring began fading into the beginnings of summer, and the third anniversary of that first surgery came and went. I was the only one aware of it (who marked it in any way). Again, I was at work. There was a day or so of melancholy, for things lost and things changed. But it passed.

That May, I celebrated my fifth year with the company. I had spent five years surrounded by books and the people who love them. We had a little ceremony and a presentation of a lovely gold-and-silver pin from Tiffany, no less! It's nice to feel like the company you work for is happy you work for them.

On the long weekend in May, I actually danced for the first time since all this began. It wasn't for long, only one song (Blondie's "Heart of Glass"). I wondered if I would ever dance again, but I was with a friend and friends of his. We had gone to The Cellblock for retro night after Bulent's housewarming party. None of the guys pressured me to dance or commented on the fact that I was just standing and watching. When the song came on and Bulent went to dance, I propped my cane against the wall, took a deep breath, and followed. It was hard. My centre of gravity was different, and my good knee ached from the extra effort of carrying all my weight. That night, I discovered I could do it. I could relearn the skill if I took the time. It didn't cause me grief to see how my ability was impaired. Over the summer, I spent more time on that dance floor, allowing that part of me come to life again.

As summer blossomed, I saw Dr. Wunder for my three year follow-up appointment. He gave me permission to stop using my cane. He said, as long as the pain and the limp weren't too bad, I could give it up. He also told the resident du jour that, when they performed the surgery on my leg, they didn't know if it was actually going to work. I'm glad I didn't know that at the time. I needed to feel they had a reasonable certainty that it was going to be fine. Their seeming confidence gave me confidence. If I had doubted the possible outcome, I think I very well might have cracked.

He also told me that it appeared the bone didn't actually attach to the prosthesis. It looked as if fibrous or scar tissue held it in place. He said it was just a byproduct of the radiation's damaging effects. The inhibited wound healing from the radiation also may have prevented the bone matrix from ossifying properly. He said the only cause for concern would be if there was pain along the joining of bone and prosthesis (there wasn't) or if there were any signs of bone loss or deterioration (there weren't). He also looked at me and said everything about my case was extraordinary.

That summer was a fun, social one. I went for coffee in patios. I spent time in bars and clubs, but not to excess and without any expectations. I met people, danced, and laughed. I felt alive again as my heart uncurled from its fetal position.

It was also the summer of the blackout, when the Eastern Seaboard was plunged into darkness on a hot August afternoon. I was at work, fielding calls from stores who hadn't realized it was a far-reaching problem or who were unsure whether to close or not. In the end, when it appeared there would be no quick resolution and our battery backup for the phones died, we made our way home.

Luckily, one of my coworkers had a car and was able to get me home through the chaotic streets. That night, I sat in the dark while candles burned in the stifling heat. I called home and let my parents know I was home and safe. I then just waited it out. I had learned that lesson well over the past few years. When there is nothing you can do, there is nothing you can do. My power was back the next morning, and the rest of the city was back up over the next few days.

That year, be it spring, summer, or fall, I saw Dr. Blackstein every six weeks, alternating chest X-rays and CTs. All continued well. But the subconscious remembers the times and places where we have been hurt and the things that have caused us pain. Even if the memories are not in our forebrain, they are still buried below the surface. As fall came again, an ambient, but growing, anxiety fell upon me. When you have been kicked enough times in a certain way, at a certain time, you become suspicious of those circumstances when they come upon you again. This was the time things had gone to hell the year before. It had occurred in approximately one-year intervals, so I was coming due again. I could feel the tension growing along my spine as I waited for the other shoe to drop. And, sure enough, it dropped again that fall.

Dr. Blackstein told me the CT had flagged another tumour in my lungs. As he said it, a frown formed on his face. The radiologist had compared it to a scan from the previous year, rendering the results suspect. Telling me it was "an indefinite maybe" (leaving me hanging in the wind), he sent me on my way and promised to let me know when a proper comparison had been done and something was known.

I grasped that faint hope and throttled it, but I knew inside it was likely to be true. I existed in a strange mix of hope and the hard knowledge that the hope was a vain one. I waited.

Once again, as my life tumbled out of balance, there was a man. I have had a history of meeting men along this journey through cancer, men I care for and seek solace from in those burning desperate hours. This time, his name was Glen. We met at The Cellblock on a Saturday night, noticing each other across the room as I waited for Nick and Rob to arrive. He looked so serious that I propped my own mouth into a smile with my fingers just to see how he would react. He chuckled. When Nick and Rob went barhopping, I stayed and danced. When I sat down, tired and sore, I caught Glen's eye. He mimicked my earlier "smile" gesture. The ice was broken.

We spent nearly twenty-four hours together and then saw each other briefly a couple nights later, just before his mother was due in town for a visit. We agreed we would meet when she returned home.

Tired of waiting, I finally called Dr. Blackstein's office and left a message. His secretary called me back promptly with an appointment to see Dr. Johnston. There was no doubt left. The shoe had dropped.

Pete offered to come with me to that appointment, and he offered to come in and listen to the news with me if that was what I wanted. I did. (Much of my reticence to ask for help has faded throughout this ordeal.) He sat beside me in another of those pastel examination rooms. This one was crammed with filing cabinets. If we had wanted, we could have read the histories of uncounted former patients. When the resident came in for the preliminary part of the meeting, we both noticed how cute he was.

Fate is sometimes a cruel bitch. This could have been a familiar procedure like the last few times. Though unpleasant, that was something I knew. But no. This tumour was in the lower left lobe, around the back. They would not be able to enter through my chest again. This would call for a thoracotomy. They would have to cut through the muscle in my back, just below my shoulder blade. Once inside, they would remove the segment the tumour was in. The procedure was called a segmentectomy. It would be a much more painful procedure.

Not only was I going through this again, it was a different procedure again. It was something unfamiliar. I couldn't rely on my previous knowledge and experience to guide me. Again, I was wandering into a strange, new territory along a different path.

After Dr. Johnston left the examining room, I hung my head and began crying, feeling utterly defeated. I was lost without any landmarks in sight or familiar constellations in the sky. Pete's hand was a tiny, diamond point of warmth and comfort on my shoulder.

When I pulled myself sufficiently together, we walked from the hospital, along College to Yonge. We then headed north. I walked blindly, not really registering anything. Pete just followed along and listened when I wanted to talk, which wasn't often. We eventually went our separate ways, and I went home. A message from Glen was waiting for me. His mother was gone. I called him back and fell apart. He asked if I wanted to come over.

I called work and let them know I wouldn't be in the next day. The rest of that week, when I wasn't working, I was at Glen's place. I hid, losing myself from the world and the reality of what was coming. But it continued to approach no matter what, so I eventually went back home and got on with the business of living as best I could.

Once again, Valerie and the team were solidly behind me. There were no worries on that count. Both Valerie and Doug, our Chief Technical Officer, were adamant I have whatever time off I needed at full pay. There was one less worry. I received messages of support from many others, including the VP of human resources. No one could ask for a better response from one's employers in such a time.

The Wednesday after that appointment with Dr. Johnston, I went to a get-together arranged by a Web site I am a member of. Mostly, I went to see a few people I am close to. Nick and Rob were there, and I told them of this latest diagnosis. Nick's face crumpled. There's no other way to describe it. Looking so lost and sad in that moment, it broke my heart. Seeing his pain at the thought of my pain gave me an insight (one of those eureka moments) into how it must have felt for any of my loved ones to have heard of my illness. Regardless of how well they covered it with hope, support, or humour, that was what their helpless anguish looked like. I put my arms around him, and we held onto each other. Then I looked him in the eye and said, "Okay, you're not allowed to be more upset about this than me!" And we laughed.

Time passed all too quickly, as it so often does when there is something we wish to avoid. It was soon time for another early morning trip to the hospital. The entourage this time included Kerry (proving to be a stalwart friend despite all of the ups and downs and horrible things I had once thought about him), Lindsay (taking time from school in London to see me safely in and out of the operating room), and Glen. Once again, we waited in the waiting room at the end of the hall on 7 Eaton South as I was weighed, had my vital signs checked, and was shaved. (This time, it was in a ridiculous pattern, from directly below my left nipple, under the midline of my chest around to the back. It was only on one side.) Due to the new post-SARS rules, when the time came to be taken to the operating room, only two people could accompany me. Glen volunteered to leave, armed with Kerry's cell number so he could check on me.

Kerry and Lindsay followed me down to the preoperative ward where we waited. One of the operating room nurses remembered me. I slipped quickly into smart-ass mode and cracked jokes to anyone who would listen. When they took me into the operating room, the table was so narrow that they had to strap me onto it. I made some comment about bondage to the anaesthetist. I can't help it. I will use humour as armour until the day I die. As Carrie Fisher wrote in her book, *The Best Awful*, "If my life wasn't funny, then it'd just be true, and that would be totally unacceptable."

The first memory I have of the recovery room is so hazy and indistinct that, if I had not seen the nice male nurse from it a couple of days later in the step-down unit, I would have sworn I had dreamed it, conjured from the drug stew in my system. There is a vague remembrance of waking in agony, feeling a pain like nothing I could describe and being rolled onto my side while they moved the epidural site in my back. Then everything went dark again.

When I woke in the step-down unit it was late, after nine o'clock in the evening. They had been running behind that morning. The surgery had started late and ended around 1:30 or 2:00. Strangely, perhaps because they doped me up so much, I slept far longer than before. Kerry and Lindsay were there. I could barely keep my eyes open. Reassured I was fine, they left me to sleep.

I didn't find out until the next day that the surgery had been more complicated than they expected. They discovered the tumour was deep and close to too many vital structures. There had not been a choice except removing the lower lobe of my left lung, about half the lung. Once again, despite the curve thrown, I had come through the surgery well without any complications.

When I regained consciousness, there was a neat, red, quarter-circle scar along my back from the inside of my shoulder blade down under my arm. Again, there were tubes and lines inserted seemingly everywhere, including the epidural, an IV, an arterial line, a catheter, and, worst of all, two chest tubes inserted between my ribs.

A quick, basic lesson: Pain is your body's way of telling you "Whatever you are doing, stop!" The more vital the part of your body is, the more sensitive to pain it is. It's your body's way of keeping those parts protected.

Your ribs encase your most vital organs. Therefore, they are extremely sensitive. Those thick, rubber tubes rubbed against my ribs every time I moved or even breathed. The pain was unbelievable.

I slept much of those first few days, frequently waking to find someone sitting beside my bed. First, there was Shawn. Mark then came with an armload of books. Then Kerry stayed. Over the course of those six days, lots of friends visited, including Lindsay, Glen, Nick, and Rob. Pete came and sat with me for nearly two hours, listening to me try to talk my way through the pain and release the gas building up inside. He just patiently waited and smiled.

In between visitors, I just lay there and waited for the time to pass and the pain to ease. The pain was so brutal and unbelievable that it had a colour, that saturated acid green that makes you squint when you see it. I spent those days riding crests and troughs of pain unlike any I had known, not even the first time they rebuilt my leg. When I was ready to go home, the pain specialist told me the epidural had been twice what it had been the previous time and they had still needed to dose me with oral painkillers to keep me from clawing myself apart.

I remember being taken to X-ray as soon as I was movable. Woozy and pained, I was sprouted with tubes. I remember hearing a cry of anguish from another patient who was also waiting, "Please, take me back. Somebody." Her tone was that of a plaintive child couched in the voice of a middle-aged woman. Perhaps mad. Perhaps only mad with fear.

Gradually, I began healing. The drainage from my lung eased as the edges began knitting together. Lines and tubes were removed one by one, and I was finally ready to go home. Glen came, bundled me up, and put me in a taxi. After a quick detour to pick up pain pills, I was home.

I spent the next six weeks slowly healing while I hobbled first around my house and then my neighbourhood. Unlike the last time, I did not have any desire to rush back to work and felt no guilt at the extra workload my coworkers were bearing. This time, my spirit was infinitely weaker than it had been last time. More time was needed to heal. I watched movies, renting them in quantity. I craved either something light and uplifting (*Bend It Like Beckham*) or mindless mayhem (*The Core*, which was fun because, as each character was introduced, I could predict the order in which they would die).

While I rested and healed, my old friend, Sandra Sprecker (she of the Avengers T-shirt) visited. She stayed with Kerry and Ken and visited to keep me company. We went for walks, had lunch, drank lattes, and talked. There is something about old friends, the ones you have known for many years. You have a short-hand drawn from a wealth of experience that lets you pick up on conversations you had years before. There is something safe about being with each other. You know each other in special ways because you have seen the changes that each has gone through. Until I saw her, I didn't realize how much I missed her.

The human body and spirit are resilient things. With me reminding myself regularly that it was all I had to accomplish, I did heal.

◆   ◆   ◆

10*28*03

The physical pain has subsided (uncounted Percocets and Tylenol 3s, not to mention two nasty withdrawals later), but I'm left with this disengaged feeling. It's like my emotions are wrapped in bubble wrap. I talked about it with my shrink. I have this strong desire to put my face out there in the media and do some volunteer work to help people facing this for the first time. I want to pass on something to people who might be helped by what I went through and what I might have learned. The shrink pointed out the unspoken motivation behind this is death, the desire to "make the most" of whatever time is left. My mortality is a constant companion these days. I take it out for tea in the long, quiet afternoons.

The doctor says this sense of noninvolvement in my own life is an understandable reaction, a sense of not wanting to "let in the clutch" because the gears will surely strip if I engage them now. The emotional healing will take more time.

◆   ◆   ◆

11*11*03

I'm going into work tomorrow to begin the process of getting back to normal, whatever that means. I want to get back to the process of living, of having a life instead of simply trying not to die. I imagine it will be like before. The first day will merely be reading e-mail and updates, trying to get some grasp on what I have missed.

I don't know how I feel about going back. It will be nice to have some structure to my days again, some place to go and something to do. The thought of the inevitable, awkward conversations—the "How are you doing?" exchanges that translate to "Please just tell me you are fine so I don't have to contemplate my mortality any more!"—freezes me. I have no idea how to explain my state of mind or body to people I respect and like, but have no training in the language of cancer.

Part of me still wants to hide from the memories of the pain and the constant struggle against the spectre of this potentially terminal illness and nurse my bruised, battered emotions and my still tender body. But I can't do that.

The first Harry Potter movie was on tonight. I found it a fitting way to bring my sojourn into recuperation to a close. Isn't it primal, that desire to be more than we are? That need to believe in magic and want that metaphorical "letter from Hogwarts" to come through our mail slot. The movie makes me tear up at the end every time I see it or reread the book. The bond of friendship and love. The responsibility to use our gifts, our "powers" for the betterment of our world. The notion that doing the right thing is rarely the easy thing.

I dislike using words like hero or bravery to describe what I went through, but I know I faced something evil, something horrible. For the most part, I kept my dignity and spirit. I didn't knuckle under, and I endured some fairly shitty stuff and managed to get through.

I think all of those comic books I read as a child stood me in good stead. They were the first place I learned those Potter-esque values. But a hero? I don't know. Besides, I look terrible in tights. But a Hogwarts robe might work…:)

◆   ◆   ◆

I went back to work on November 12, managing to read through 395 e-mails before giving out and heading for home. That day, I tried cramming as much information into my brain as I could and get a feel for what's been happening. It was good to see everyone again. It all felt mostly normal. But hearts and minds scar more easily than flesh and take longer to mesh together again.

◆   ◆   ◆

11*19*03

There are days when the ground falls away from under my feet, leaving me on a precipice, dangerously unbalanced. Beneath me yawn the many shades of hell that have ruled my life for the last three-plus years. Every horrible moment of my cancer combines and kicks me in the gut, and I just want to take to my bed. I sometimes wonder if this is what Vietnam vets feel, this post-traumatic stress disorder. The feeling creeps up on you. Nothing will ever be good again.

The triggers can be something benign. Today it was the rain, bringing the sinus headache as the barometric pressure shifts along with it. Sometimes, it is a taste, a smell, or some trigger that reminds me of all they did to me. Sometimes, it is the new aches and pains that permeate my flesh. The ache in my rebuilt leg because I need new shoes. Or there is this residual tenderness along the left side of my rib cage or the tightness along the new scar on my back after a day at work. Or there is just the plain, old stupidity of dating and trying to forge a connection with another man in some meaningful way that might last.

I know this feeling is transitory, and I will feel better in the morning. But I sometimes wonder if, even though the fissure will seal and leave my footing more secure, the damage runs too deep. I wonder if my feet may not give way under me, but I will never really soar again.

◆   ◆   ◆

Through almost everything that has happened in my life, I have been blessed with being functionally dysfunctional. I may be cracked and bleeding on the inside, but I can still get up on time, get to work, and do my job. The ability to function, to appear normal, is a great survival tool. Taking one of my old acting teacher's words to heart ("Fake it 'til you make it!"), I continued acting as if things were normal and fine. The more normal I pretended to be, the more normal I felt. I had my follow-up appointment with Dr. Johnston and received the pathology report: surgical margins (clean), bone sample (clean); lymph nodes (clean). At work, we pushed on to Christmas.

Twenty-Two
Way Beyond Empty

My sister Jennifer has been here for the last few days. She's on her way to Montreal for a conference. It's been nice. On Saturday, we went for brunch with Tanya and Gordon. We then went out to the Beaches. In the evening, we watched the two X-men movies because she had never seen them. Today, we went to the ROM. In between, we watched TV, ate, and relaxed.

It's been normal. The cancer hasn't come up as more than a passing reference in the context of some other conversation. In a way, I'm almost grateful it happened offstage for my family. We can do all the ordinary things we usually do together without the taint of treatment, surgery, or anything else. I can dissect the experience here with my friends who saw it up close and these entries and my book. I can keep my family life safe from the blood, vomit, and pain. The times when we manage to be together, those moments of jaw-dropping insanity when the world makes no sense at all, are very far away.

◆　　　◆　　　◆

My next hospital appointment would be on December 9. It was time for both my six-week follow-up appointment with Dr. Blackstein and my six-month follow-up appointment with Dr. Wunder. With Dr. Blackstein, everything was fine. He just went over the pathology report with me and said we might even be able to reduce the frequency of our appointments.

I went for leg X-rays and then saw Dr. Wunder. He took my leg and held the thigh. He then took the ankle and moved it from side to side to check how much play there was in the prosthesis. The expression on his face told me before the words came out of his mouth.

◆　　　◆　　　◆

12*09*03

Way beyond empty inside
Awaiting my last day to arrive
Way beyond empty inside
Awaiting my end to arrive.
—Lyric by Zakk Wylde

The bushing in my prosthetic is starting to go. If it isn't fixed, the metal ends will begin grinding against each other. There will be metal residue in my system, and there is a very real possibility that the shaft could break where it's embedded in the bone.

The replacement will involve a couple days in the hospital and maybe another Zimmer splint until the incisions heals. It's nothing major, just a tune-up. My head knows it will be a minor procedure. So why do I feel like the world is ending? I'm so tired, numbed, and broken down by this constant struggle against this disease. I can't even feel my life anymore. I can't feel the life I fought so hard to keep. Everything is an inch away, behind a slab of plate glass.

For the first time since this began, I think I feel despair. I wish the cancer had just killed me three years ago, once and for all.

◆　　◆　　◆

That night, I came home, closed the door to my room, and cranked the music. I played Concrete Blonde and Evanescence as loud as I could stand. (If you ever hear me listening to Concrete Blonde, you know I am pissed, especially a song called "Heal It Up.") I sang until my voice hurt. (Have you ever wanted to scream so loud that your vocal chords would tear?) I stayed there and turned in on myself.

Months later, Gordon took me to task in his gentle way for making it hard for him to approach and help me with the feeling, for hiding my pain once again. What he didn't understand is that there are sometimes words too horrible to speak aloud. Words that will tear and burn our mouths if we utter them, if we give them voice and make them true. I couldn't say those words yet.

The next morning, I told him as I was preparing breakfast and getting ready for work.

◆　　◆　　◆

12*10*03

Why has this path been laid before me? Why has this happened? I know it's pointless to ask, and there's no answer anyway, but my heart is so wounded. It has all played out in such perfect horror that, if it had been carefully scripted, it couldn't have hurt me more.

Just when I had reached a point that I could accept the possibility of not going through another lung surgery if I got sick again, the bushing goes in my knee. It's nothing life threatening. It's just inconvenient and serious enough to be dealt with. I have no real choice.

Then I meet men who seem interested in me, who hesitate to say or do anything and then meet someone else and fall in love. I almost meet someone who becomes a dear friend and feel kinship with, but he feels no desire for me. I meet someone who loves me and who I feel safe and comfortable with, but he's married. There are any number of other emotional tortures to compound this growing despair in my heart.

The fates have slipped those knives in deep and perfect, knowing just how to hurt me the most. All I want is for someone to hold me while I cry and keep the demons away for a short time. But I can't even feel my life anymore.

◆　　　◆　　　◆

I feel I should make a distinction here, even though to some it might not seem like much of one. In those days, I was in no danger of swallowing pills or slitting my wrists. It wasn't that I wanted to die. I just wished, when the cancer had first come, it had been terminal and spared me the intervening years. It was a retroactive death wish, not a current one. In facing this illness, I have had to face my mortality. The thought of dying holds little fear for me anymore. I'm not eager to leave this world, but, when my time comes, it comes. I have reached a place where I honestly believe there are things worse than death and things that frighten me more. But life has a way of rolling on and sweeping us along in its current, regardless of what changes we wish for.

◆　　　◆　　　◆

12*12*03

I had dinner with my niece Wendy tonight. She was in town for work, and we were able to connect. We haven't seen each other in ages. Like all of my relationships with my family, it's like no time has passed. I've missed her and her husband, Don. It seems, by the time we really recognized each other as people, as fully fleshed adults, we had moved to different cities and led separate lives.

It helped to see her, to just sit in that familiar pattern of family and talk about my feelings and the experience of my illness with someone who is permanent, who I have known almost since birth. She is someone who really understands me because we sprang from the same genetic stock.

I was talking to an online acquaintance today about how I fear that my feelings are just scarring over. I had to make myself so strong to survive this experience that I may just eventually not feel anything. How disturbed I am that I can't even cry. He was trying to help, but, in the end, I just logged off without saying good-bye because he was just pissing me off so much and missing how I felt completely.

The sense of utter loss and despair has faded a bit. It's amazing how the patterns and the habits of smiling, laughing, and being "normal" slip into place to keep one going. But I still feel angry, lost, and in need of something I can't even begin to name, let alone ask for. I look into the faces of my new friends and see they are trying to help, but I just want to scream "No, that's not it! You don't understand. That's not what I'm asking you for!" I can't seem to translate the language of cancer to English.

◆　　　◆　　　◆

12*17*03

The tension is easing somewhat. I've been busy at work as we ramp up for Christmas, so I haven't been given a lot of brooding time.

My last few entries have upset my sisters. As my new friend Ron says, the feelings have to be expressed if they are authentic. And that is true. We spend so much time denying how we feel that we are scared, angry, and bereft. We need to speak about those feelings and bare them to the light. It is the first step to confronting them, understanding them, and moving beyond them.

This is my path. For some reason, the universe has decided this is where I must go. It sucks, and it's brutal, but I am here. And there is something I must yet do. I know what it is. Now, all I have to do is figure out how to make it happen and just endure these setbacks when they happen.

I have met some amazing people in the last three years, whom I have grown to love a lot. Sandra, Lindsay, Martin, Peter, Nick, Rob, Mike, and Glen. Every medical professional who has helped me. The people I work with now. There has been richness amid the devastation.

It's foolish to think that one somehow affects the other; the meeting of these people eases the pain of the illness and makes it all worthwhile. The gain of one does not take away from the loss of the other. But I love them all, and they will see me through if it is at all possible. That much I know.

◆   ◆   ◆

Christmas that year at work was crazy with all sorts of things going wrong, but I was amazed at how well we all handled it, from the support team to the people in our stores. I had only a little time off over the holidays, but that was fine. I have grown accustomed to working over the holidays, and I stocked up on DVDs and made myself a nice dinner on Christmas Day. The only person I saw was Pete, who came over for a hot chocolate. I made tentative plans to go home once things calmed down in 2004.

Glen had gone home for the holidays, but the cracks were already beginning to show. Days went by without phone calls either way. I knew the end was coming.

I say this with neither pride nor shame, but these short-lived flings characterized my whole journey through my illness. As the boom fell each time, I met a nice man and attached to him, needing the comfort that being with someone would bring. But, once the crisis passed, the surgery was over, and the healing had begun, I would see the things that made me not want to be with him any more. Or I would equate him with the ugliness that had occurred and be unable to face the associations that came with him. I don't know what the mix was with Glen, but it just fell away. Like I said, I'm not ashamed of myself. I wish I had handled things better in many cases, not just with the men in my life. But I didn't. And I will live with my mistakes and the knowledge I have hurt people. And I will try to learn.

That January, Kerry and Ken moved to England. They had wanted to go for about a year, and a wonderful opportunity came up for Ken that made it perfect for them to go. I was happy for them, but the pangs ran deep. There was an abiding feeling that, while Kerry's life had improved, mine had worsened. It's hard watching someone who used to be with you having dreams come true while you are fighting for your life. But comparing yourself with others doesn't lead one anywhere. His path was his, and mine was mine. It took me a while to get here, but I'm glad he's doing well.

When the surgery date came, it was a surprising bolt from the blue. Barbara, Dr. Wunder's secretary, phoned on Monday, January 19. The surgery would happen that Friday. Because there was no time for preadmission, I would be admitted on Thursday afternoon and be ready the following morning.

This time, I would travel to the hospital alone, splurging on a cab. Pete would come the next morning in time for the surgery and be the contact who would pass along the news when I came out of the operating room.

That week, my emotional life was a sine wave, careening from peace to terror, a kind of baby bipolar. There was a sense of dread that something terrible was waiting, but it alternated with a sense I was at least on familiar ground again and the hospital was the safest place to be.

I entered Mount Sinai that afternoon on an Ativan high without any worries. I was comfortable in that place as soon as I walked through the door. But the trough hit after dinner as visiting hours ticked away. I told Pete that visiting hours ended at nine o'clock, forgetting the post-SARS changes. Visiting hours actually ended at eight o'clock, and I had no idea how strict they would be. Each passing minute brought me closer to not seeing my anchor, my good friend whose duty was just to show up to keep me from fear. Thankfully, Pete arrived just before eight o'clock and stayed for an hour or so.

The man in the next bed cut our visit short. Ninety-one years old, he was in pain from the most recent of four hip replacements in the course of two years. The pain medication confused him. One moment, he was politely asking me to help him find his glasses. The next, he was sharp and bitter at Pete and me for talking and accusing me of not going to bed at 9:15. I turned out every light except one, closed the door, and hunched over my book on my rolling table.

"Isn't this a hospital room?" my roommate kept asking. Finally, I gave up and went into the lounge across the hall, biting my tongue against my anger. He is old and in pain. I can relate to at least the latter half of that. But I bristled. Perhaps the reason he made me so angry was because I saw my possible future in him, old and weak after endless surgery and treatments, lost in a forest of pain and fear I have already been in for far too long.

◆   ◆   ◆

01*23*04

The morning of the surgery, I am deep in sleep when the nurse wakes me. As I drag myself awake, panic thuds in my stomach. Why does time pass so quickly? It's too soon!

Once again, I am in the control freak's worst nightmare, the ultimate loss of control. Waiting in the dark to be drugged, manipulated, and cut up once again. Butterflies in the stomach become boulders.

I dread going into that dreamless dark. The last thing I remember before unconsciousness sets in is the bright and cold. Then I come to in that moment of utter disorientation, returning from sleep changed or with some piece of myself gone.

◆   ◆   ◆

I actually did dream that time. Or I at least remember dreaming that time just before I woke in the recovery room. I don't remember what, just the soft, cloudy feeling quickly replaced by a rending, taffy ooze as the real world broke through. It was like swimming to the surface of a swimming pool through water made thick and syrupy.

What Dr. Wunder had thought was a blown bushing was actually something different. The femoral stem held by fibrous tissue instead of bone had come loose. That was the source of the side-to-side play he had felt in the leg. He had replaced the femoral stem, cemented it in place, and replaced the bushing for good measure. When I saw him, I could read in his face that he was happy with how things had gone. It didn't really surprise him what had happened. The procedure had taken about as long as he had originally estimated for the bushing replacement, around four hours.

I was back in the same place I had been almost four years before, a thick Jones bandage on my leg with the incision held together by staples. I was tubed and cathetered once more.

I have mentioned this state of having foreign things entering my body at various orifices before, but I can't stress enough how annoyingly complicated it is and how unpleasant it is. You cannot move without tangling something or pulling at a tube or needle or line that is inserted into your flesh or, in the case of a catheter, your urethra. (Despite what certain fetishists may tell you, that is a place nothing should ever be inserted!)

The Saturday following my surgery, after he had a terrible afternoon of painful muscle spasms, the man who had angered me a couple days earlier slipped into confusion from the pain pills he had been given. He lay there, raving and moaning. They tried taking his blood, but his veins were too small and weak. As he grew more agitated, I felt myself tensing. I understood how he must have felt, but he argued, moaned, and complained when the nurses told him what to do.

The next day, the physiotherapist, Becky, came to my room with her assistant, Andy. As on my last time, the first step was the high walker and the manipulation of tubes to get them out of the way. Becky supported my bandaged leg, and I made it out of bed into the walker.

A dull bloom of pain went through my knee. I couldn't keep weight on it, so they propped me in a chair and left me to sit up for a while. Ten minutes later, I became dizzy, not uncommon for being upright the first time. I broke into a cold sweat all over my body. My vision began blurring, and bright smears of light obscured the room. I buzzed for help getting back into bed, but I could hear Becky talking to another patient in the hall. No one came for what seemed an eternity, but it was merely five minutes or so in real time. I buzzed again, and Andy came through the door almost simultaneously. Becky followed with Yoi, the nurse. Once I was in bed, they checked my blood pressure and oxygen saturation, which had both dropped sharply. The feeling began passing, and I felt better.

There were tears that came and went for a long while afterwards. Once again, it would be harder than I thought. Once more, the problem was actually more serious than the doctor thought. Once more, the hospital stay would be longer, and the recovery would be more difficult. When Yoi, my nurse, saw my tears, she said, "Don't be hard on yourself. That happens to a lot of people." I tried explaining the feeling. I wasn't upset with myself, just the circumstances and the constant uphill battle to get well. I don't know if she understood. Once again, I struggled to translate.

◆   ◆   ◆

01*25*04

Time stretches, bends, and ceases to mean anything. I have to really think to recall what day it is. I don't know if I can do this again. But, even that feeling has become déjà vu because I have felt it going into the last three surgeries. I've been sure, no matter what, I couldn't do it again. But, when the time came, I presented my plate for a fresh serving of hell.

Am I just some sort of masochist? Is there some need in me to keep on subjecting myself to this torture? Or is it just the deep-seated drive to endure, to hang on and survive? Maybe it's just still that "best little boy in the world" thing that tells me I must be strong and keep going. Perhaps I just can't let the cancer win. I am just fulfilling the "I don't think so" promise (threat) I made to it when all of this started.

◆   ◆   ◆

When Dana, the physiotherapist working on Monday, saw me, the Jones bandage had been removed and the incision looked good. It was stapled cleanly and healing.

We fit my Zimmer splint, battered and stained from my last go-round, onto my knee. She supported my leg and helped me to stand into the walker. With her support, I slowly put weight onto my newly mended leg.

There was no pain. I felt some pressure along the incisions and awkwardness from the splint, but no pain. I walked out of the room to the first cross corridor, a journey much like the one I had taken nearly four years earlier. Then I went back to my room and into a chair while Sandy, my nurse that day, finished changing my bed. I sat. Without prompting from Dana, I hooked my good foot under my bad leg and used it to lift the bad leg onto the stool as Andrea had taught me the first time around. Dana was surprised I knew how, but the body remembers.

Sitting there, for the first time in a long time, I felt something like a small triumph, something like hope, which had become somewhat of a stranger in my house of late. At that moment, I could actually believe this would be easier this time, the road might get better.

My panic and tears the previous day had been premature. The road did get easier. The next day, the physiotherapist had me go up and down a flight of stairs. It was simple. It was the same process I had been using all along since the first surgery. When going up, lift your weight with the good leg. When going down, lower your weight onto the bad leg and drop the good leg to meet it. This was something I knew, something I had mastered long before. Other than the awkwardness of having my leg splinted, I could move around well. The physiotherapist said, "You graduate."

On January 28, with all tubes and such removed, Pete picked me up at 8:00 AM. I truly had come full circle. It was a morning diametrically opposed to the sunny morning in June, four years earlier, when I first exited the hospital. It was grey and snowy with dirty, slushy drifts lining every street from the two-day blizzard a couple days earlier, but one thing—the most important thing—was the same. I was out.

Twenty-Three
Me...Now

One of the random notes I scribbled in my little book says that cancer stories don't really end. Even if you are one of the lucky ones and your cancer is cured, the effects continue to be felt. It is such a profoundly life-changing experience that it can't help but stay with you forever.

I was not one of the lucky ones in that respect. The experience kept repeating, taking much longer than I expected. Even now, there are no guarantees it is over. I no longer think in terms of being cured. I have learned to enjoy the idea of being in remission and hope the remission lasts a long time. But, if it comes back, I will fight again. I know I can do that.

I have written the ending to this book three times. Unlike my illness and my life, this book cannot continue indefinitely. In the same way I had to choose an arbitrary point to begin the story, I must choose another one to end it.

The last time I rewrote this, I had just had the staples removed from my leg. The incisions healed well and with very little pain. Initially, I had lost nearly all of my range of motion, and I thought it would mean months of hard physiotherapy again to get it back. But the gods smiled on me in that respect. My knee loosened up in the week I waited for my appointment. When my range of bend was measured, it was seventy degrees and, with a bit of effort, eighty. Now, I am back to almost ninety on my good days.

For the first half day, I was happy. Then I found myself growing angry and suspicious as if it was all some practical joke, like someone would jump out, yell surprise, and take it all away. Four years of disappointments and getting smacked down just as I am pulling myself back up have left their mark. But I am not at the mercy of those feelings, and I am getting better at accepting this bit of good fortune.

Much has changed in the time since that last surgery. When a better job became available, I applied for it and was promoted. Now, I write and design communications for a living with the same company that has nurtured me through all of this. I took up painting big, bold canvases that relax me when it seems very little else can. The nicest thing is the self-critical voice that once kept a running tally of the things I was doing wrong in my art has gone silent.

My checkups have remained clear. I finally managed to make it to my one-year anniversary cancer-free. There was a scare before Christmas that left me wondering and worrying for a couple months, but it proved to be a false alarm. For the first time, an expectation of bad news was not borne out. It made for a welcome change.

Even this new road through health has not been easy. In the summer of 2004, I took a bad step, and my knee buckled. I had a bad fall, and the memory of that last surgery was still so fresh and vivid that I managed to work myself up into such a panic that I went into shock and passed out. I then spent almost eight hours in the emergency room waiting to be checked out. The erosions that run through me run deep, even now. I have learned my disability is a fluid thing, one that changes with the weather, my exertions, or the shoes I wear. It is different all the time. I am using my cane again.

At the core of my being, I have come to terms with many things. I have made many mistakes in my life. My finances are a disaster, and my love life is not much better. But I made peace with what I have and have not done with my life when I prepared myself for the possibility of not surviving. Everything from this day forward is garnish. For the first time in a long time, I feel like this might just possibly be over.

That faith and feeling of hope scares me, even disturbs me a little. I have hoped before this was over and was sorely disappointed. As the cancer was strong and held onto me with a fierce grip, the urge to hope is strong as well. The desire to believe a state of "all right" actually exists is powerful in me. I was afraid of pain, but I made peace with it. I was afraid of dying, but I made peace with the possibility. I have made peace with this yearning to hope and allow myself to believe, if even only a little.

I'm not saying things are perfect. I have a streak of anger in me that wasn't there before. I am more impatient than I once was. Thankfully, these remain an inside voice, a monologue in my brain when people piss me off.

I still often experience strange anxiety reactions. When SARS hit Toronto, I was getting over a cold and took my temperature obsessively for several days. One time, when I was home in Saskatchewan, I had a weird nervousness about travelling on the highway with my father at the wheel, which is patently absurd. My father is a better driver in his seventies than many are in their twenties.

I'm still being watched very closely. When I finally reached my one-year anniversary of my last lung surgery without any recurrence, Dr. Blackstein reduced the frequency of my visits from every six weeks to every three months. The occasion was momentous.

Every time I go though, there is something in the air. It's not fear. I don't think I fear this much anymore. It's an expectation, a charge in the air like ozone before a storm. There is a certain knowledge this might be another of those cusp moments that could change everything. There is nothing to do except wait until the crash happens. As I write this, I have been in remission for twenty-one months.

Several months ago, Dr. Blackstein said they wouldn't let up on the monitoring for a year. If I can make it that long without a recurrence, they will ease up—slightly. The magic number is five years. Sarcomas are one of the types of cancer that, if you make it to five years, the probability of recurrence goes down so radically that you are considered cured. But Dr. Blackstein has seen synovial sarcomas recur twenty years later. There are many years of watching over my shoulder ahead.

I said to Jon Hunter once that the hardest thing was finding a balance. We have to plan and build as if we have a future, yet love and live as if we don't. We have to learn to carry the ghosts with us and learn to listen to them, but we don't give them too much power when they whisper in our ears. It's like the day I was waiting for the streetcar, and I put the plastic holder holding my Metropass in my mouth as I needed my hands. As soon as my teeth clenched on it, I felt my gag reflex start to go. I think it was a combination of the act of clenching my teeth (as I had done in those spates of vomiting) combined with the smell of the plastic (like the little blue basin I vomited into). The body never forgets.

My body has become a catalogue of new aches and pains in the places where the cancer once was and in the spaces it once filled. There is the dull, constant rub of flesh against metal in my knee every time it is bent or straightened, every time I sit or stand, or even sit or stand too long in one position. There are the pokes in my good knee (it feels strange to call it that, as if the prosthesis or "bad" knee is somehow just mischievous or ill-behaved) as it lifts my body weight climbing stairs or rising from a seat. There are the aches, sometimes sharp, along my sternum, where it has been sawed open twice. There is the pull of the scarred flesh and muscle along my shoulder blade that bites when I slouch or don't sit properly. There is the contradiction Jon Hunter told me of once. Translated from French, it is the "painful numbness" (which you will recognize when you feel it) along the lower ribs on my left side and along my left leg where there is nerve damage. My big toe, immobile after the first surgery, regained its mobility, though that foot feels as if someone is gripping it tightly on hot days. When I breathe deeply, I can feel the absence of the lower half of my lung, as the intake of air is lopsided, stopping several inches short of the limit on my right side.

I have grown accustomed to these strange sensations, these times of pain. It never really goes away, but it offers a constant reminder of what came before. When it comes, it is an old friend, a travelling companion. We know each other well. We know each other's ways and each other's quirks. Its power over me has lessened when I learned to accept it as a fact, as one of the foundations my life is built on. It is there, but it is like a radio playing in another room. (For a fascinating look into pain, read *Pain: the Science and Culture of Why We Hurt* by Marni Jackson.)

I am dating again and not taking it too seriously. I've met some nice men and some utter wing nuts. I still want to fall in love again and settle down, but it isn't the burning need it used to be. It's more like wanting to skydive or see Paris. It would add something to the flavour of my life. Without it, I am whole, and my life is okay. I am past forty now. I don't think anyone can look at the prospect of living life solo and not feel twinges. It becomes a different kind of game in midlife. Still, my life is full and well lived. I've made some new friends who look out for me, make me laugh, and remind me that I'm still here.

I still can't really grasp the concept that I am walking on eighteen inches of metal or half of my left lung is gone. The idea is still strange and science fiction-y. It is there in the front of my brain, but it's not really in my soul yet. I wonder if it will ever be.

In the course of all my appointments, scans, and surgeries, I have developed a love/hate relationship with hospitals. At times, my stomach churns before I go in, anticipating the pain and the humiliation, the gowns and IVs, and the constant interruptions for pills and vital signs. Perhaps even more, they represent another lapse, another misstep into the land of cancer.

I also find hospitals familiar and strangely safe. I know their secrets. (I know the easiest way to get to the upper floors of Mount Sinai is taking the back elevators on Murray Street.) I know, for all the things I hate, hospitals have healed me and pulled me back from the awful pit of illness. Whenever I have to go for a follow-up or an appointment with Jon, even for the most recent surgery when Dr. Wunder repaired my leg, as soon as I walk through the doors, I feel a surge of calm and peace that whispers, "This is familiar. This is safe."

After it all, I'm tired—physically, emotionally, and spiritually spent. It's more than I have ever been in my life. These last two surgeries took much out of me and left me shell-shocked and broken. This disease has both made and unmade me. I feel as if I have become a walking quantum uncertainty, like Schrodinger's cat waiting for the box to be opened. When it happens, the wave function will collapse. I will either fall in love again, or I won't. I will either get sick again, or I won't. I will either survive it, or I won't. In the weak moments, which have grown more frequent as the four years of illness progressed, when I am exhausted or in more pain than usual or lonely for a lover's touch, I give in and wish the disease had taken me. Those feelings are pit stops, just a momentary skid of the wheels on glare ice. In the end, they are just emotions. There is no way to go back in time and change what has occurred. This has been my path, and I can only accept it and walk it to the best of my ability.

For the most part, perversely, I am happy. I like where I live and what I do. I feel safe in the love of my friends and family. Even in the face of uncertainty, I feel a sense of tranquillity most of the time. I've never thought of happiness as an emotion. Rather, it is a direction, a choice. It is a decision to be made. An acquaintance told me recently that the reason I survived was because I just love being here so much. Though I had never thought of it in those terms, it's true.

I feel like I've turned a corner. It's like the transition phase has ended, and the actual new life has begun. It's the life of my new, altered body. It's the life of me with my sometimes painful, often stiff knee. It's the life with the cane and dramatic scar. It's the life of the second chance I was granted, whether that second chance lasts a month, year, or lifetime. Again, it's a lifetime of "I'm not going to die, now what?"

With every part of my being, I hope this is the end. Or, at the very least, it will be a good long time before I have to face this again. I hope my strength will see me through again and another recurrence won't be the straw that broke the camel's back. I hope these loving, wonderful friends will continue holding me up and keep me going when I lose my way.

Like the wash of headlights on a dark road at night, there is only so much we can see. The rest is blackness, and we will only see what waits in the darkness when we come upon it. We discover the path as we walk it.

So, I take a step. My left leg swings forward, and my foot comes down. The prosthesis locks into place, and my footing is solid. The pain is not so bad, so I take another and another. Right...left...right...left...

And breathe.

Acknowledgments

It is said that a true friend knows the song in your heart and can sing it back to you when you forget the words. On those days when I forgot this song, Mark Lefebvre was always there to remind me of the melody. Thank you, my friend.

In terms of putting the package together, thanks go to Peter Mitchell for his fine-tooth comb editing; Steve Gaydos and Richard Stoltenberg for their cover design inspirations; Debra Marshall for the front cover photograph; and David Findlay for the back cover author photo.

Much gratitude to Heather Reisman for gracing my cover with her generous quote and to everyone at Indigo for keeping a place open for me, giving me the chance to grow, and helping me get this on the shelf.

Thanks to gifted writers and unofficial mentors Robert J. Sawyer, Suzanne North, and Nalo Hopkinson for gracing me with such glowing words of praise. You inspire me every day.

Eternal gratitude to the three graces, my sisters Susan Brooks, Linda King, and Jennifer Saemann, who charged to the rescue and kept me believing when I wasn't able. Also to my family—every niece and nephew, aunt, uncle, and cousin, every great, grand aunt twice removed who kept a fire burning in their hearts.

To my beautiful friends, too numerous to name, for throwing out the lifeline when I needed it most and holding on tight.

And last—there are too many to name here—to every doctor, nurse, physiotherapist, and radiation therapist who was there to take care of me, I thank you with everything I am yet to be. I am here to write this because of you.

Suggested Reading

When I was diagnosed, the first thing I did was go to the Health section of my store and get books to read. If you need to read more about cancer, here are some titles courtesy of Indigo's Trusted Advisor Program, Canada's source for expert book recommendations from Canada's leading physicians and healthcare professionals:

- *Choices*, by Marion Morra and Eve Potts, Harper Collins Canada, (0060521244)

- *Facing Cancer: A Complete Guide for People with Cancer, Their Families, and Caregivers*, by Mikkael Sekeres and Theodore Stern, McGraw-Hill Canada (0071414916)

- *Coping With Chemotherapy and Radiation Therapy* by Daniel Cukier, Frank Gingerelli, Grace Makari-Judson, and Virginia McCullough, Mcgraw Hill Canada (0071444729)

- *Mayo Clinic Guide To Women's Cancers* by Charles Loprinzi, Kensington Publishing Corporation (189300533X)

Knowledge is your first weapon against cancer. These should give you a place to start and the list of titles on the Trusted Advisor list is always being updated. Check for more at www.indigohealth.ca

978-0-595-37530-1
0-595-37530-8